Healthy Foods, Healthy Kids

Also by Elizabeth M. Ward
Pregnancy Nutrition: Good Health for You and Your Baby
Super Nutrition After 50 (coauthor)

Healthy Foods, Healthy Kids

A complete guide
to nutrition for
children from birth
to six years old

Elizabeth M. Ward, M.S., R.D.

Adams Media Corporation
Avon, Massachusetts

Published by Adams Media Corporation
57 Littlefield Street, Avon, MA 02322. U.S.A.
www.adamsmedia.com

ISBN: 1-58062-595-9

Printed in the Canada

J I H G F E D C B A

Library of Congress Cataloging-in-Publication Data
Ward, Elizabeth.
Healthy foods, healthy kids: a complete guide to nutrition for
children from birth to six years old / by Elizabeth Ward.
p.   cm.
Includes index.
ISBN: 1-58062-595-9
1. Children--Nutrition. 2. Diet therapy for children. I. Title.

RJ206 .W278   2002
613.2'083--dc21   2001055306

This publication is designed to provide accurate and authoritative information
with regard to the subject matter covered. It is sold with the understanding that the
publisher is not engaged in rendering legal, accounting, or other professional advice.
If legal advice or other expert assistance is required, the services of a competent
professional person should be sought.
— From a *Declaration of Principles* jointly adopted by a
Committee of the American Bar Association
and a Committee of Publishers and Associations

Cover photograph by: Stephen Simpson/FPG International
Additional interior photographs ©2002 Medela Inc. Used with permission
of Medela, Inc., McHenry, IL.
Quiz on pages 133–4 reprinted by permission of the American Dietetic
Association.

This book is available for quantity discounts for bulk purchases.
For information call 1-800-872-5627.

Visit our home page at *www.adamsmedia.com*

For my family.
You make it all possible.

CONTENTS

ACKNOWLEDGMENTS

Writing is a solitary business, yet I am not solely responsible for this book. I had help.

I especially want to thank friends who reviewed the manuscript for me, pointing out areas for improvement and making the book better for its readers. They include Cindy Carroll, M.S., R.D., who provided speedy feedback and who has supported me throughout the writing process, and Sheah Rarback, M.S., R.D., a pediatrics expert. I worked through many of the ideas in the book with Hillary Wright, M.S., R.D., and our pediatrician, Howard Rashba, M.D. I appreciate their time and expertise.

My encouraging husband and my three daughters inspired me more than they will ever know as I worked on *Healthy Foods, Healthy Kids*. They are the reason I write.

Chapter

A

Learning

Experience

Mom, how do
you know what
to feed us?

—Hayley, *age five*

The answer to this question from my oldest daughter may seem obvious. After all, I am a registered dietitian with a degree in human nutrition and fifteen years of experience in the field. That's only part of the reason why I have an edge on feeding my family, however. Without question, my profession makes it easier for me to choose and prepare nutritious foods for my daughters. But nothing beats parenthood as a proving ground.

It wasn't until I became a mother for the first time, nearly six years ago, that I began to understand the rigors and the joys of feeding young children on a daily basis. Years of on-the-job training with three children ages five and under has softened my rigid notions of how kids should eat—ideas that I freely dispensed in my pre-kid days.

Hands-on experience has brought an unexpected renewal of professional passion, sparking an interest in how eating right sets the stage for a child's future health and well-being. It's rewarding to see the positive effects of a balanced diet unfold before you as your children fill out and get taller, begin to crawl and then walk, and learn to read and write. As a mother and a dietitian, it's gratifying to know that instilling healthy eating habits at an early age will help reduce my daughters' risk for chronic conditions such as cancer, osteoporosis, and heart disease later in life.

You may think that being a dietitian provides immunity to the challenges of feeding three youngsters. If only that were true! Like all parents, my husband and I struggle with getting the kids to eat nourishing meals and snacks. In spite of our best efforts, our daughters favor a limited number of foods. They'd rather dine on boxed macaroni and cheese or store-bought chicken nuggets, French fries, and ketchup (that's a vegetable, right?) than anything else. And our youngest prefers drinking her calories as milk and juice rather than consuming them in the form of solid food. Not exactly what I had in mind.

HOW TO USE THIS BOOK

As a loving caregiver, you want to nourish your infant, toddler, or preschooler in the best possible way, which includes providing him with a well-balanced diet that supplies the nutrients he needs to maximize his physical and intellectual development.

Like so many other parenting skills, choosing the right foods, dealing with picky eaters, and juggling the nutrient needs of an entire family is a learn-as-you-go proposition, and one that is in constant flux.

Parents often ask me how I handle myriad feeding issues with my own children, which is why I have included so many personal experiences in *Healthy Foods, Healthy Kids*. But this book is not designed to preach the virtues of my way of raising children as the only way. Rather, it's meant to supply practical facts and solid advice so that you will feel more confident feeding your little tike from infancy until the day you send him off to first grade. *Healthy Foods, Healthy Kids* is packed with anecdotes, tried-and-true eating tips and techniques, and a wealth of nutrition information every parent or caregiver of young children should have at their fingertips.

So when your breastfed baby has trouble taking a bottle and you are days away from returning to work, when your daughter turns up her nose at the tuna casserole she's loved for months, or when your five-year-old son has a tantrum because you've nixed his request for a sixth cookie, turn to *Healthy Foods, Healthy Kids* to help you formulate feeding strategies that work for you and your family.

Not Mini-Adults

To get a sense for how much nutrient needs vary between adults and children, consider the requirements of a thirty-seven-year-old mom and her six-month-old son.

At first glance, it seems that mom needs more nutrients than her baby, but very young children are far more needy than their parents. Comparing nutrient needs based on body weight puts into perspective baby's high nutritional requirements. The daily quotas for the select nutrients listed here are much lower for the infant, but only because he is smaller. In reality, on a pound-per-pound basis, baby needs triple the calories, about two and half times as much protein, more than five times the vitamin C, and four and a half times the iron. In addition, fat should contribute upwards of 50 percent of an infant's calorie intake, whereas the adult recommendation is 30 percent or fewer fat calories.

Suggested Daily Requirements

Age/Weight	Calories	Protein	Vitamin C	Iron
6 months/13 pounds	650	13 grams	30 milligrams	6 milligrams
37 years/138 pounds	2200	50 grams	60 milligrams	15 milligrams

ALIKE, ONLY DIFFERENT: WHAT YOU MUST KNOW ABOUT CHILDREN

In chatting with other mothers about feeding youngsters, I hear of challenges similar to my own, as well as about other "food fights" that haven't yet cropped up in our household.

Many of the moms I've spoken with take pains not to impose adult eating standards on their children, which in many ways is a wise move. Why? Your children may look like smaller versions of their mom and dad, but they are not miniature adults when it comes to nutrition. You are full-grown, so your nutrient needs are relatively fixed. But your child's dietary requirements fluctuate with age.

A child's rapid development translates into tremendous nutrient demands. Infants in particular go through a mind-boggling growth spurt during their first twelve months. Full-term babies without health problems typically double their birth weight by five months and triple it by their first birthday. Toddlers and preschoolers don't grow as quickly but do steadily gain weight and get taller with the passing years.

Health experts say that during a child's first formative years, too much of any one nutrient can be as harmful as too little. That's why adult dietary recommendations usually don't apply to a youngster's diet. For example:

- The National Cancer Institute recommends 20 to 35 grams of dietary fiber every day for people over age eighteen, but a child's fiber requirement is linked to his age. That explains why a four-year-old needs less than half the fiber of an adult. Getting more fiber than she needs on a regular basis may do more harm than good. Why? Fiber is filling. A child's small stomach capacity means she may not have the room to finish higher-calorie foods that are necessary to fuel her growth. In addition, excess dietary fiber can cause diarrhea.

- Mom or Dad may need to reduce fat intake to lower elevated blood cholesterol concentration or for weight control, but it doesn't pay to curb fat in a very young child's diet. The reason: Restricting fat can stunt brain development as well as overall growth in children under the age of two.

- Certain foods are simply not fit for a very young child. Giving milk to infants is a good example. You may be trying to include three glasses of milk every day, but pediatricians say feeding regular cow's milk to infants instead of iron-fortified formula or breast milk threatens their development; serving reduced-fat milk in any form before age two may hamper growth, too.

PUT NUTRITION TO THE TEST

How do you decide what foods to eat and what to serve to your little one? Your meal and snack choices are shaped by several factors, including past food experiences, personal food preferences, and nutrition knowledge.

The more nutrition facts you have at your fingertips, the easier it is to feed your family a healthy diet. The following quiz can help you find out how much you know about nutrition. Don't worry if you don't ace the test. It's by no means exhaustive, and it's intended to highlight areas where you need additional information. After each answer, you'll find a reference to the part of *Healthy Foods, Healthy Kids* that sheds more light on the issue; this feature is particularly helpful when you come up with the wrong answer, but also beneficial for learning more even when you answer correctly.

1. Fiber provides 4 calories per gram.
2. Kids can outgrow their milk allergy.
3. Starting solid foods will help your infant sleep through the night.
4. When your baby doesn't finish drinking all of the formula in his bottle, you should discard what remains.
5. Sugar causes hyperactivity.
6. It's OK to restrict dietary cholesterol in kids, no matter what their age.
7. Osteoporosis, the brittle bone disease often responsible for fractures in older adults, actually begins in childhood.
8. Saturated fat contains more calories than monounsaturated or polyunsaturated fat.
9. Children need juice every day.
10. Nursing mothers need more calories than pregnant women.

Answers:

1. **False.** Even though fiber provides calories, humans cannot make use of it. That's because fiber passes through our digestive system nearly almost intact. So why is fiber so important for kids and adults? See page 16 to discover fiber's role in a child's diet.
2. **True.** Even though cow's milk is the most common cause of allergic reactions in kids, most children outgrow the problem by the time they celebrate their fourth birthday. What's more, true food allergies are relatively rare occurrences, affecting only about 2 percent of adults and 5 percent of children. Refer to Chapter 12 for more information on food allergies.

3. **False.** It would be nice if all it took for Mom and Dad to get a good night's sleep was a bit of baby cereal. But it's not so. According to the American Academy of Pediatrics (AAP), babies sleep for extended periods only when their digestive and nervous systems are developmentally ready to do so. That's why feeding baby the likes of baby cereal and pureed vegetables cannot discourage her night owl tendencies, especially if she's only a few months old. Plus, health professionals frown upon introducing solid foods before four months because baby's digestive system is not yet mature enough to process it. Learn more about introducing solid foods on page 98.

4. **True.** Reusing the formula or milk left over in baby's bottle is asking for tummy trouble. Bacteria from baby's mouth makes its way into the fluid where it can reproduce to proportions that could cause intestinal upset, even when the remaining liquid is refrigerated. While it may rub you the wrong way to toss unused formula or milk, better safe than sorry. One way to avoid waste: Serve baby smaller portions. Check out other food safety tips in Chapter 11.

5. **False.** The power surge toddlers and preschool-age children get from eating sugary foods is only temporary. It is not at the root of hyperactivity, a chronic condition characterized in part by inattention and impulsiveness. It may be irritating when kids act wild after munching on candy, cakes, and cookies, but nutrition experts maintain sugar has no long-term effect on a child's ability to learn or to concentrate. That's not to say that you shouldn't limit sugar, however. Sugar is explained in detail beginning on page 13.

6. **False.** While the National Cholesterol Education Program recommends that everyone over the age of two consume 300 or fewer milligrams of cholesterol per day, there are no suggested limits for children younger than two. Cholesterol is key for brain development and should not be kept from infants and young toddlers. More often than not, cholesterol is found in fatty foods such as whole milk, meat, and cheese. Restricting fatty foods curbs cholesterol consumption, but it can also compromise growth. Fat is a concentrated energy source that young children need to fuel their rapid development. Check out cholesterol starting on page 24.

7. **True.** It may be a condition of the aged, but when it comes to dietary factors, osteoporosis goes back to what you ate throughout your lifetime, beginning in childhood. Youth is a time of rapid bone formation, a period when the body is most keen on absorbing calcium from foods and laying it down in bones to shore them up for later on. A poor diet, especially one

lacking in the bone-building nutrients calcium and vitamin D, puts kids at risk for hip fractures decades later in their fifties, sixties, seventies, and eighties. Find out more about calcium and bone health on page 28.

8. **False.** All fats contain the same number of calories, nine per gram. From a health standpoint, the difference between them has largely to do with their effect on blood cholesterol levels. Excessive amounts of saturated fat (greater than 10 percent of your total calorie intake) may boost blood cholesterol concentrations like no other element in the diet, at least in adults. The unsaturated varieties of fat are far more artery-friendly; they don't promote the clogged blood vessels that can lead to heart attack or stroke. Facts about fat begin on page 21.

9. **False.** While six ounces of juice counts as a serving from the Food Guide Pyramid's Fruit Group, kids don't need to drink juice for good health. Pure fruit juice is a good source of several nutrients, including potassium; many are even fortified with calcium and vitamin C, adding further benefit. Yet, juice is devoid of fiber. And sipping too much juice may translate into weight gain, even in active children. In fact, drinking excessive amounts of juice may make for a shorter child. Discover more juicy facts on page 41.

10. **True.** Lactation requires that you eat an additional 500 calories a day, whereas pregnancy boosts daily calorie needs by 300. The suggested calorie intake for breastfeeding accounts for the fact that, during pregnancy, your body stores fat that can serve to nourish the baby in addition to the extra 500 calories you eat daily. Find out all the particulars of what nursing women should eat beginning on page 80.

Chapter 2

Nutrients That Matter Most for Kids

Nutrition is really important to me. I want my kids to be strong, successful, and healthy, and good food is a big part of that.

—Laurie, mother of three

THE ENERGY PRODUCERS

Most children are so energetic that you can get tuckered out just trying to keep up with them. Toddlers learning to walk, run, and climb and preschoolers who flit from one activity to the next all day without stopping seem to have boundless energy reserves. There's probably not a parent on this planet who hasn't marveled at his or her child's energy level.

For all the running around they do in a day, it's amazing that a mere three nutrients provide kids with the fuel they require to learn, play, and grow. The body harnesses the calories in the carbohydrate, fat, and protein found in food and converts them into the chemical energy that runs all bodily functions.

Counting on Calories

Without adequate energy, kids cannot develop to their fullest potential, physically or intellectually. How many calories your child needs is really up to her. Why? Because every child has unique energy requirements. That makes the following chart with figures from the Food and Nutrition Board of the National Academy of Sciences more of a guideline than a rule for calorie consumption. So don't worry if your child's calorie intake doesn't match up exactly to the figures below. As long as your pediatrician says your child is growing fine, then she is eating enough.

Suggested Daily Calorie Intake

Age	Weight (lb)	Height (in)	Calories
Birth to 6 months	13	24	650
6 months to 1 year	20	28	850
1 to 3 years	29	35	1,300
4 to 6 years	44	44	1,800

CARBOHYDRATE, THE PREFERRED FUEL

The body favors carbohydrate as an energy source. At 9 calories per gram, fat has more than twice the calories of carbohydrate, which provides 4 per gram. But the body has an easier time of using carbohydrate to meet its constant energy demands.

Eating adequate carbohydrate spares protein to do its important work. Protein can provide as many calories as carbohydrate, but when the body employs it as an energy source, protein is diverted from its more important functions, including providing the raw materials for the frantic cell production taking place in your child's growing body.

To prevent the body from using protein for fuel, carbohydrates must dominate the diet. When it comes to children over the age of one, about 50 to 60 percent of their calories should come from the likes of breads, grains, cereals, fruits, vegetables, beans, and dairy products. Infants need more fat, however. During the first year of life, babies require only about 40 to 55 percent of their calories as carbohydrate.

Simple, Yet Complex

Carbohydrates are categorized as simple sugars or complex carbohydrates. With the exception of fiber, each gram of carbohydrate provides 4 calories. Fiber is a complex carbohydrate, but since humans cannot break down fiber in their digestive tract, we can't use the energy it would otherwise provide. Nevertheless, fiber is necessary for both children and adults (see "Fiber," page 16).

Nutrition experts say foods rich in complex carbohydrate are the healthiest for every family member and should be the main source of carbohydrate calories. Foods packed with complex carbohydrate, such as starch, typically contain other vital nutrients, are generally low in fat and cholesterol, and are fiber-rich. For example, fortified whole grain breads and cereals contribute complex carbohydrate and fiber; B vitamins, including folic acid; and iron nutrients that everyone, particularly kids, needs for good health.

Simple sugars, including table sugar (sucrose), fructose, maltose, dextrose, honey, molasses, maple syrup, corn syrup, and brown sugar, are sweeter than their complex counterparts. Most parents are concerned about their child's simple sugar consumption, and with good reason. By and large, sugar-laden choices serve up little in the way of good nutrition. Sugary foods, including cookies, cakes, and candy, supply calories that kids need to grow, often with few other attributes. That's why it's no surprise that studies show that children who more often choose sweet, low-nutrient fare over foods such as milk, fruit, and whole grains, come up short for several vitamins and minerals as well as for fiber.

How Sweet, and Healthy, It Is

It's important to note that fructose is a major component of most fruits, and that lactose, also a simple sugar, is the primary carbohydrate in milk and milk products. (Simple sugars, including sucrose and corn syrup, are typically added to dairy foods such as yogurt, chocolate milk, and frozen desserts, hiking the carbohydrate content.) Yet, there is no reason to eliminate milk, yogurt, cheese, and cottage cheese because of their simple sugar content; nor should your child avoid fruit.

In fact, fruit and dairy foods make excellent substitutes for more processed sweet snack choices, including pastry. Fruit offers vitamins, minerals, fiber, and phytochemicals, plant substances that scientists say may ward off chronic conditions such as cancer and heart disease; these nutrients are missing from cookies, cake, and candy. When kids sip small portions of orange juice mixed with club soda or seltzer water in place of soda, they benefit from the nutrients, most notably vitamin C, that soda and many other sugary beverages lack. All the better when the orange juice is fortified with calcium, since calcium-added orange juice typically provides as much calcium as milk.

In My Experience
Don't Go Overboard

Curbing a child's consumption of sugary foods is a wise health move. However, I've found that keeping kids completely away from soda, candy, and cookies actually backfires in the long run. Scientific research bolsters informal observations of my patients and of my own children. A study published in the *American Journal of Clinical Nutrition* suggests that while restricting a child's access to his favorite foods is appealing to parents, it only makes kids want them more. The researchers concluded that trying to keep kids away from their favorite fare is not effective when trying to promote a moderate intake.

MYTHS AND FACTS ABOUT SUGAR

Myth: Sugar Causes Hyperactivity in Children

Fact: When your child bounces around like a Ping-Pong ball after eating the likes of candy, cake, and cookies, it's typically a short-term energy surge. There is no evidence that sugar by itself can turn a child with a normal attention span into a hyperactive one. Researchers say studies suggest sugar has no long-term effect on a child's ability to learn or to concentrate and that eating sugar does not cause hyperactivity, a condition characterized by impulsiveness, inattention, distraction, and anxiety.

If the truth about sugar is hard to swallow when your child is going bonkers, consider this: caffeine could be culpable. Colas, with the exception of the caffeine-free varieties, can provide a prolonged power surge for little bodies, but so can certain non-cola drinks that contain caffeine, including Mountain Dew and iced tea. And don't forget that kids often consume sweet foods in highly charged social situations such as family gatherings, birthday parties, and holiday celebrations. For more facts on caffeine, see page 40.

Myth: Sugar Makes Kids Fat

Fact: No single nutrient is to blame for weight gain. All calories count toward energy balance, including those from protein, fat, and all forms of calorie-containing carbohydrate.

The major problem with sugar is that it can sneak into everyday foods, increasing their calorie count. That means children consume more calories without eating additional food. Here's how it works. When your child adds 3 level teaspoons of sugar to his low-sugar breakfast cereal, he piles on 48 extra calories. That may not sound like a lot, but over the course of a year, it adds up to 17,520 calories, the equivalent of about five pounds of body fat.

Certain sugar-laden foods such as chocolate and donuts are also rich in fat, which is part of the reason for their extreme calorie counts. For example, a commercially prepared pecan roll can easily supply 800 calories and 45 grams of fat. It also packs the equivalent of more than 10 level teaspoons of sugar. In this case, fat contributes 50 percent of the total calories, while the sugar provides 20 percent.

Regular physical activity—often in short supply in a child's lifestyle—helps to counteract excess calories in any form.

Myth: Sugar Causes Diabetes

Fact: Diabetes is a hereditary condition. It's unclear what triggers type 1 diabetes, the most commonly occurring form in children, and the type that requires daily insulin injections for life. Experts say viral infections, exposure to toxins, and emotional stress may "turn on" the gene for diabetes in children. Children with a parent or sibling with type 1 diabetes should avoid cow's milk for their first year of life to reduce the chances of developing this variety of diabetes.

Myth: Only Sugary Foods Cause Cavities

Fact: Sugary foods up the risk for developing cavities, but so does eating any form of carbohydrate, with the exception of fiber.

Foods filled with starches, such as whole wheat breads and cereals, are actually no better for your child's teeth than sugary foods. That's because the mouth harbors carbohydrate-craving germs that form a sticky film called plaque. Mouth bacteria thrive equally well on the sugars and starches found in fruits, breads, cereals, grains, and sugary beverages. As bacteria feast on carbohydrate, they produce acid that makes holes in a tooth's enamel, its protective outer coating. Sugary foods are particularly problematic because they can linger on teeth, promoting acid production long after eating is over. Each time you consume carbohydrate in any form, acid from mouth bacteria attack your teeth for at least twenty minutes. Encouraging children to brush twice daily with fluoride toothpaste and eliminating frequent snacking on foods rich in carbohydrate, including juice and soda, help curb cavities.

SUGAR REDUCING TIPS

There's no harm in small doses of sugar, as long as your child's diet is otherwise healthy. Even children with diabetes can figure in some sugar with the help of a registered dietitian. Here's how to provide maximum nutrition with minimum sugar.

- Serve sugary foods along with or after a well-balanced meal or snack such as a grilled cheese or peanut butter sandwich on whole grain bread, vegetables and dip, and milk. Food in the stomach slows down the body's absorption of sugar into the bloodstream, keeping kids' energy level on a more even keel.
- Can the soda and offer milk, water, or small amounts of fruit juice mixed with seltzer water instead.
- Make your own chocolate milk by adding one teaspoon chocolate syrup to eight ounces of milk. The homemade version offers all the benefits of milk with less sugar than commercial varieties.
- Bake with less sugar. Unless a quick bread or muffin recipe is already designed to be lower in sugar, you can use one-quarter to one-third less sugar than the recipe calls for.
- Keep candy out of sight to prevent kids from snacking on sugary foods at will. For snacks, dole out cheese or a mixture of pretzels, whole grain cereal such as Chex, and mini melba toasts or pieces of bagel chips. Kids over the age of four may munch on nuts, popcorn, whole grapes, and raw vegetables instead of candy, but these foods are hazardous for younger children as they can cause choking.
- When kids can't brush, have them swish water in their mouth to wash away carbohydrate; older children can get the same effect by chewing sugarless gum.
- Stay away from sweetened yogurt unless it's a brand that tends to use less

sugar, such as Stonyfield Farm. Low-fat fruit-flavored yogurt typically contains the equivalent of 6 level teaspoons of added sugar. Use less sugar by making your own sweetened yogurt at home. Start with plain yogurt and add a teaspoon of jam, jelly, molasses, or honey (no honey for kids under age one). Stir in crunchy whole grain cereal to increase complex carbohydrate and fiber content.

- Purchase plainer cookies such as graham crackers and fig bars, which also contain fiber as an added boon.
- Instead of a full bowl of sugary cereal, mix a child's high-sugar favorite with a brand containing little added sugar, such as Cheerios or Multi-Grain Chex.
- Top low-sugar cereals with berries, dried fruit, or sliced bananas instead of sugar.
- Opt for plain oatmeal instead of instant oatmeal in packets (it contains lots of added sugar and it costs more, too). Add chopped apple, pear, dried cranberries, or raisins to oatmeal to provide the bulk of the sweetness.
- Dip strawberries, dried fruit, or banana chunks in melted dipping chocolate and serve to children instead of candy.

No Honey for Your Sweetie

Never feed honey in any form (even in baked goods) to a child under the age of one. Honey may contain heat-resistant, toxin-producing spores of *Clostridium botulinum*, a bacteria that causes infant botulism, which can be fatal. After one year of age, the digestive tract begins to mature to the point where the health threat from honey is diminished, which is why experts say it's OK to give honey to older kids.

FIBER: COMPLEX, YET SIMPLE

You may know it as roughage, but did you know that fiber is a complex carbohydrate like no other? It is often described as the part of plant foods such as grains, vegetables, and fruits that cannot be fully digested by humans. The fact that we cannot completely break down fiber in the digestive tract sets it apart from its complex carbohydrate counterparts, including starch.

There are actually two kinds of fiber in food, soluble and insoluble. Soluble fiber dissolves in water. Despite the technical distinction, health experts do not discern between the two when making eating recommendations.

Fiber: The Benefits

Fiber contributes no calories to the diet, even though it's critical to your child's health and should be a part of his or her daily eating regimen. Why all the interest in a food substance that passes through the body largely intact? Several reasons.

Like other complex carbohydrates, fiber keeps good company. It's found in foods packed with vitamins, minerals, and phytochemicals, which are protective plant compounds.

Dietary fiber and fluid work together to prevent constipation in adults and in little ones. Fiber absorbs many times its weight in fluid. Sipping adequate amounts of water, milk, and juice enhances fiber's ability to soften stools and to add bulk, which stimulates the intestines to pass waste faster and with greater ease.

Keeping constipation out of your child's life may seem like a matter of comfort. But there are other reasons to pass regular stools. Experts say laxation, regular bowel movements, may mean that any potential carcinogens in the stool (probably from foods) will have less time to interact with the tissue of the intestinal tract, thereby decreasing colon cancer risk. A bulkier, easier-to-pass stool also dilutes carcinogen content.

Fiber may also curb the chances of developing heart disease, type 2 diabetes, and other digestive disorders, such as diverticular disease, that occur much later in life. Researchers are unclear on the effects of a high-fiber diet beginning in childhood, but they suspect that fiber is protective in the long run.

Since fibrous foods are more filling, a high-fiber diet often makes for easier weight control. Studies suggest that obesity, which is more common than ever among American preschoolers, is less likely in populations that consume a diet rich in complex carbohydrate and fiber. That makes sense. Highly-refined foods, such as white bread, corn flakes, and candy, are not as satisfying as higher-fiber choices. Fiber-rich foods fill you up so that you eat less. For example, your child may find it difficult to down 250 calories worth of fiber-rich bananas (about two and a half pieces of medium fruit) because of their bulk, but have no problem nibbling the same number of calories as fiber-free milk chocolate (the amount in a small candy bar).

Fiber: The Downside

While fiber's ability to fill you up is a boon to adults watching their waistlines, it's actually a pitfall for children.

Kids have such small stomachs that too many servings of whole grain cereal and high-fiber fruits and vegetables can jeopardize their growth. Fiber-filled foods can crowd out the higher-calorie fare children need in order to grow. The situation is made worse when the overall diet is very low in fat, which is the most concentrated calorie source. In addition, high-fiber diets in children and in adults may reduce the absorption of the minerals iron, zinc, and calcium.

Figuring Fiber

Adults (those over eighteen years of age) require between 20 and 35 grams of dietary fiber every day, no matter what their age. But children are different. The American Health Foundation has come up with an easy-to-use method for gauging how much fiber children ages three through eighteen should eat. To figure daily fiber needs in grams, add the number five to your child's age. For instance, a three-year-old requires 8 grams of daily fiber, while your six-year-old should aim for 11 grams every day.

Focus on Fiber

You know how much fiber your youngster over the age of three needs. Use the Nutrition Facts panel on food products and this list of high-fiber foods in kid-size portions to help kids meet their daily quota.

Food	Fiber (Grams)	Food	Fiber (Grams)
Pear, with skin, 1 medium	4	Potato, ½ medium, baked, with skin	2
Figs, 2 dried	4	Sweet potato, ½ medium, baked, with skin	2
Garbanzo beans, ¼ cup	3	Whole wheat bread, 1 slice*	2
Bran flakes, ½ cup*	3	Kidney beans, ¼ cup, cooked	1.5
Raisin bran, ½ cup*	3	Banana, ½ medium	1
Apple, with skin, 1 medium	3	Broccoli, ¼ cup, cooked	1
Pumpernickel bread, 1 slice	3	Peas, ¼ cup, cooked	1
Oatmeal, ¾ cup, cooked	3	Tomato, ½ medium, raw	1
Orange, 1 medium	3	Brown rice, ¼ cup, cooked	1
Strawberries, ½ cup	2		
Lentils, ¼ cup, cooked	2		
Carrots, 1 medium, raw	2		

*Check Nutrition Facts label for exact amounts; they vary by brand.

LOW-CALORIE SWEETENERS: OK FOR KIDS?

Your child loves sweets, and you'd like to give him more sweet foods. Too many naturally occurring simple sugars in the likes of soda, candy, and cookies, and the threat of obesity and cavities makes it tempting to serve children foods sweetened with low-calorie alternatives such as aspartame, saccharin, acesulfame-K, and sucralose. With the exception of aspartame, which contains a few calories, these four sweeteners approved for use in the United States are calorie-free and none of them contribute to tooth decay.

You may benefit from judicious use of reduced-sugar foods as part of a balanced diet, but I don't recommend them for your child. Why not? Youngsters require a variety of fresh and lightly processed foods to thrive. Highly processed fare sweetened with low-calorie agents does not have a role in a diet that promotes proper growth and development unless a youngster has diabetes or another condition that precludes him from eating simple sugars without consequence. Chances are, if you think your child would do better by eating foods with low-calorie sweeteners, you should probably rethink his diet.

Powerful Protein

Carbohydrate may be the energy workhorse, but no nutrient beats protein for providing the raw materials for rapid growth and development.

Each gram of food protein provides 4 calories. But we eat protein-packed foods primarily for their amino acids, not for their potential energy. Amino acids are the building blocks of the protein found in foods, as well as body proteins. During digestion, protein is broken down to amino acids, which the body uses to construct the likes of neurotransmitters for brain function, cells, muscle, skin, hair, and the hormones and enzymes that control your child's bodily functions.

Protein: Meet the Need

Protein requirements steadily decline in relationship to body weight as your child matures. As long as your breastfed or bottle-fed baby is eating enough, you probably have little to worry about on the protein front. As children make the transition to eating more solid foods and drinking less formula or breast milk, you may see a dropoff in protein intake, but that doesn't mean they aren't getting enough. Here are estimates of kids' protein requirements, and foods that help satisfy them.

Age	Daily Protein Requirement (grams)
0–6 months	13
6–12 months	14
1–3 years	16
4–6 years	24

Protein Amounts

Food	Protein (grams)	Food	Protein (grams)
Formula, 1 liter (33 ounces)	14–16	Peanut butter, 1 tablespoon	5
Breast milk, 1 liter (33 ounces)	10	Macaroni and cheese, ½ cup, prepared	5
Pork, top loin, 1 ounce, broiled	9	Tofu, ¼ cup, raw	5
Chicken, 1 ounce, roasted	9	Soy beverage, 4 ounces	5
Canned tuna, white, drained, 1 ounce	8	Milk, 4 ounces	
		Whole	4
		1% low-fat	4
Beef, extra lean, 1 ounce, roasted	8	Yogurt, 4 ounces	
		Whole milk, plain	4
Pizza, cheese, 2 ounce slice	8	Low-fat, fruited	4
		Bread, whole wheat, 1 slice	3
Cheese, cheddar, 1 ounce	7	Bulgur, ½ cup, cooked	3
Cottage cheese, ¼ cup	7	Garbanzo beans, ¼ cup, cooked	3
Chicken nuggets, 1 ounce, cooked	6		
Egg, 1 large, whole	6	Pasta, enriched, ½ cup, cooked	3
Lentils, ¼ cup, cooked	5		

Strike the Right Protein Balance

Protein is an important part of everyone's diet, but it is particularly paramount for young children. Here's why. Amino acids prompt the body to build proteins during periods of growth, fostering peak development of brain and body. Since she cannot store amino acids, your child needs a fairly steady supply. Consuming protein at regular intervals throughout the day helps meet your child's amino acid demands.

Quality Counts

Amino acids are not created equal. Your body can make twelve of the amino acids needed for good health, but the other nine must come from food. *Essential amino acids* (EAAs) is the term given to the nine amino acids the body is incapable of producing. While the other twelve have been deemed nonessential amino acids (NEAAs), they are no less important to your child.

Animal and plant foods both supply amino acids, but with a difference. The protein in animal foods such as eggs, meat, seafood, and dairy products provides all, or nearly all, of the EAAs your child needs. Plant foods, including rice and beans, contain fewer EAAs, and no single plant food contains every EAA. That's why people who avoid animal foods entirely (including dairy and eggs) must eat a wide variety of plant foods daily to get the full complement of EAAs the body requires. The amino acid pattern in breast milk is considered ideal for children one year and under.

While the quality of protein (i.e., its amino acid profile) is crucial to everybody, getting adequate amounts of EAAs means even more to a youngster. That's because kids require more of the EAAs to fuel their rapid growth. Skimping on protein-packed foods means leaving out NEAAs, too. A child's body can make the NEAAs that are missing from a protein-deficient diet, but that conversion comes with a price: Making your own NEAAs uses up precious calories, and prolonged calorie deficits could limit your child's growth.

FOCUS ON FAT

It's not a four-letter word, but it might as well be. Fat is despised by adults for its ability to pack on the pounds and, depending on the type, to boost blood cholesterol levels.

True, fat can hamper weight control. You may avoid it because each gram provides 9 calories, more than twice the amount in carbohydrate or protein. Its calorie count is a boon for children, however. Satisfying their elevated energy demands would be next to impossible with just carbohydrate and protein. In fact, fat is so critical to growth that experts recommend an infant's diet derive half of its calories from fat. Breast milk supplies the right fat in the right amounts and changes over time to meet the needs of a developing infant. Adults are most often advised to limit fat calories to 30 percent or less of their total energy intake.

Fat is much more than a source of energy:

- The body, especially a growing one, needs the fat in food for the essential fatty acids (EFAs) it provides. Like EAAs, EFAs cannot be manufactured by the body and must be provided by food. EFAs are the raw materials for building cells, particularly those in the brain.
- Fat plays a monumental role in brain development. A detailed discussion of how fat fosters brain function begins on page 56.
- Fat helps dissolve and transport vitamins A, D, E, and K, which are necessary for your child's bodily functions. In addition, fat provides satisfaction and makes food taste good by providing flavor and texture.

Good Fat/Bad Fat

All three types of fat provide the same number of calories but act differently on blood cholesterol level, affecting your heart disease risk. Despite the fact that we tend to categorize foods according to the type of fat they supply, foods are actually a mixture of the different fat types. For example, olive oil is mainly unsaturated fat, yet it contains 14 percent saturated fat by weight. That's why experts recommend eating small amounts of the healthiest fatty foods, such as olive and canola oils.

Saturated fat raises blood cholesterol levels like no other food component. Animal foods, including full-fat dairy products, butter, fatty cuts of meat, certain processed meats such as bologna and salami, poultry skin and fat, and lard ,supply saturated fat. Palm oil, cocoa butter, and coconut oil used in processed foods such as cookies, crackers, candy, and snack chips contain concentrated amounts of saturated fat, too.

Trans fats are similar to saturated fats in their health effects: They, too, boost blood cholesterol levels when eaten in excess, even though scientists don't agree about which fat is worse for you. The hydrogenated vegetable oils found in margarine, shortenings, and other processed foods are particularly rich in trans fats. Some commercially fried foods such as fast food chicken nuggets, French fries, seafood, and bakery goods, including scones, pastry, and apple pie, pack trans fats, too. Right now, you won't find trans fat content listed on the Nutrition Facts label. Because trans fats are similar to saturated fat, the Food and Drug Administration (FDA) has proposed that trans fatty acids be lumped into saturated fat content on food labels.

Unsaturated fats, including the polyunsaturated and monounsaturated varieties, help keep cholesterol concentrations in check as part of a diet that is low in total fat content. Unsaturated fats are found in vegetable oils such as olive, canola, and corn; nuts, including peanuts, cashews, and almonds; and avocados. Fish, particularly the fattier ocean species such as salmon and bluefish, harbors an unsaturated fat called omega-3, which is particularly useful to your child's developing brain. See page 57 for more on the omega-3 fat docosahexaenoic acid (DHA).

How Low Should Children Go?

Excess fat promotes obesity. Too much saturated fat and trans fatty acids increase heart disease risk. The detrimental effects of fat serve as the basis for the argument to limit fat intake. But do fat restrictions apply to your young child?

Yes, and no. The suggestion to curb fat intake is directed at children two years of age and above, as well as at adults. According to several health organizations, children should begin the gradual transition to eating less fat at age two and strive for limiting fat to 30 percent of total calories by their fifth birthday.

That's certainly sound advice, but it can be misconstrued. Although parents are advised to begin feeding kids a diet lower in fat at age two, that does not mean that it's beneficial to begin before that time. In fact, it's harmful. A low-fat diet during infancy and early childhood is typically short on calories and nutrients, particularly the brain-building fats (DHA) and arachidonic acid (AA), which are critical to a child's peak development and vision. The AAP says older children should consume a minimum of 20 percent of their calories from fat. Yet, there is no reason to be super strict on fat intake, even in three, four, and five-year-olds. One report published in *Pediatrics* found that kids who ate less than 30 percent fat calories lacked adequate energy, calcium, iron, and protein, while their counterparts consuming 40 percent or more fat calories did not. That's not to say a higher fat diet is necessarily a healthier one, however.

So what's a parent to do? Even though researchers say that a lifelong preference for lower-fat foods probably begins in childhood, you don't need to make a big deal about fat. The suggestion to limit fat does not mean that every food in a child's diet must be low in fat or devoid of it. Eating too many calories from any source, including carbohydrate and protein, will also foster weight gain when not balanced by physical activity.

Balancing some high-fat selections with low-fat fare typically goes a long way toward good health. Rather than trying to get a four-year-old to understand the concept of a balanced fat intake, provide her with a variety of foods, and let her choose for herself. For instance, a meal of homemade chicken nuggets, carrot sticks and salad dressing for dipping, a roll with margarine, and 1 percent low-fat milk provides a mixture of high- and low-fat fare. When it comes to treats or desserts, serve up graham crackers, fresh fruit, and reduced-fat frozen yogurt more often than ice cream or candy, but don't feel you should leave out the latter.

In My Experience
I'll Take the Real Thing—Most of the Time

There's no fat-free margarine, fake-fat snack chips, or light cookies in my kitchen. The only reduced-fat foods we use with any regularity are milk and yogurt (our youngest still gets whole milk dairy products because she's under two). Why do I shy away from the bulk of commercially prepared lower fat foods? It's largely lack of nutritional merit. In many cases, when you take the fat out of the cookies, crackers, and peanut butter, you must replace it with sugar or other carbohydrates (or water or air, in the case of margarine) or sodium to make it edible. Much of the time, products end up lower in fat but not appreciably lower in calories. And because they lack fat, you may actually eat more of them, defeating the original purpose, which I suppose is better health.

CLEARING UP CHOLESTEROL CONCERNS

Most people curse cholesterol, but you need it for life. Cholesterol is a fatty waxlike substance that every body makes, even your little tike's. In fact, the myelin surrounding your child's developing nerve cells is composed of 15 percent cholesterol. The increased need for fat and cholesterol is why pediatricians recommend a high-fat diet until age two.

Cholesterol is required for digesting and absorbing the fat from foods, as well as for producing hormones, the bodily substances that orchestrate the functioning of organs and tissues. In addition, cholesterol is part of cell membranes, serving to protect the inner workings of your child's cells. It's also the raw material for the production of vitamin D, necessary for bone strength.

If cholesterol is so great, why all the bad press? Because cholesterol in food is perceived as public enemy number one when it comes to clogging arteries. But that reputation is not well deserved. Studies show that the saturated fat in food raises blood cholesterol concentrations with much more force than does dietary cholesterol.

BEHIND THE SCENES: VITAMINS AND MINERALS

Carbohydrate, protein, and fat may garner the most attention, but they would be nothing without the vitamins and minerals that support them. Vitamins and minerals do not provide energy for youngsters or adults, but they direct the metabolism, digestion, and absorption of the three energy-producing nutrients. Minerals in particular orchestrate bodily functions that often involve carbohydrate, protein, and fat. Minerals are also part of bodily structures: calcium lends strength to bones and teeth, while iron helps ferry oxygen as part of red blood cells.

It's unnecessary to count every microgram, milligram, or International Unit of the vitamins and minerals in your child's food in order for him to get enough. Vitamins and minerals are found in varying levels in an array of foods, which is one of the many reasons why nutritionists preach variety. Children who eat adequate amounts of different healthy foods have the greatest chance of meeting their nutrient needs.

While many vitamins and minerals are crucial to a child's development, they are too numerous to mention in detail. Here are the most important ones, and why.

Vitamins

Vitamins are either fat- or water-soluble, meaning they dissolve in, and are transported by, fat or water. Fat-soluble vitamins—A, D, E, and K—are stored in your child's liver and fat tissue, but the water-soluble ones—the B vitamins and vitamin C—are not. That means that children and adults require the B vitamins and vitamin C every day. Even though it's important to consume enough of the fat-soluble vitamins A, D, E, and K on a daily basis, falling short for a few days won't make much of a difference because your body has reserves of these nutrients tucked away in tissue to be used as needed. When it comes to vitamins and minerals, just because a little is good does not mean a lot is better. This is especially true of the fat-soluble vitamins: Excessive amounts over time can overload the liver and damage it.

Fat-Soluble Vitamins

Vitamin A

Role in the diet. You may remember it as the key to good vision, but vitamin A does much more than make for healthy eyesight. It's a nutrient that gets around: Vitamin A is necessary for the growth and development of all cells in your child's body.

Food sources. Vitamin A comes in two forms: retinol and carotenoids. Retinol is found in animal foods such as fortified milk and liver. Plant foods contain carotenoids, which the body converts to vitamin A on an as-needed basis. Breast milk and formula provide adequate vitamin A for infants.

Excellent vitamin A sources include:

- Sweet potato
- Carrots
- Spinach
- Winter squash
- Cantaloupe
- Tomatoes and tomato products

Vitamin D

Role in the body. How many times did your mother tell you to go out and play? Little did she know that the sunshine was setting you up for stronger bones. Strong summer sunlight sparks the production of vitamin D in your skin, a process that's finished off in the liver and kidneys. Vitamin D promotes the uptake of calcium from foods and helps deposit it into bones and teeth where it provides strength that lasts for decades to come.

Food sources. Commercial infant formulas provide adequate vitamin D, but breast milk is low in this vital vitamin and could be even lower when mom avoids milk. That's why the AAP says that vitamin D supplements may be necessary for breastfed infants, particularly those who are not regularly exposed to sunlight, who have dark skin, and who are dressed heavily when they do go outside. Ask your pediatrician whether your infant qualifies for supplemental vitamin D. Ironically, sunshine beats food as the best vitamin D source. Few foods are naturally rich in vitamin D, but there are some good sources:

- Egg yolks
- Milk (most milk is fortified with vitamin D, but read the label)
- Fortified margarine, cereals, breads, infant formula

Vitamin E

Role in the body. Vitamin E is a cellular bodyguard. It wards off the damage done by free radicals, destructive forms of oxygen that rove the body looking to stir up trouble by oxidizing cell matter. In acting as an antioxidant, vitamin E prevents anemia and preserves nerve tissue. In the long run, preliminary studies suggest a role for vitamin E in warding off heart disease and cataracts, one of the leading causes of blindness in older adults.

Food sources. Certain fatty foods are the richest vitamin E sources going, which argues against very low fat diets for young children. Common cooking oils, including olive and canola oils, contain concentrated amounts of vitamin E. Excellent sources include:

- Wheat germ cereal
- Nuts and nut butters, most notably almonds
- Sunflower seeds (a choking hazard for kids under four)
- Avocado
- Mayonnaise

Vitamin K

Role in the body. Vitamin K is necessary for proper blood clotting. Soon after your baby was born, he or she received a vitamin K injection to prevent a common bleeding disorder in newborns. Vitamin K is also involved in bone health by promoting the activation of osteocalcin, a bone protein that must be fully formed for bone strength.

Food sources. Here are some top vitamin K picks.

- Romaine lettuce
- Broccoli
- Spinach
- Egg yolks

Water-Soluble Vitamins

The B Vitamins

The B vitamins may be viewed as a group of nutrients with similar functions. Nearly all are necessary for releasing the energy from food and helping your child's body use it properly. Thiamin (B_1), riboflavin (B_2), niacin (B_3), vitamin B_6 (also known as pyridoxine), folate (also called folic acid), vitamin B_{12}, pantothenic acid, and biotin are part of the B-complex group. Here's a brief overview of how "the Bs" help children thrive.

B Vitamin	Function	Food Sources
Thiamin	Metabolism of carbohydrate, fat, and protein.	Pork; enriched, fortified, and whole grains; legumes
Riboflavin	Metabolism of carbohydrate, fat, protein, and the B vitamins niacin and B_6.	Dairy products, whole and enriched grains, whole eggs, broccoli
Vitamin B_6	Metabolism of carbohydrate, fat, protein, and niacin. Prevents anemia; promotes a healthy immune system.	Meat, poultry, fish, bananas soybeans, garbanzo beans
Vitamin B_{12}	Healthy nervous system and heart. Prevents anemia.	Beef, lamb, canned tuna and salmon, milk, fortified milk, soy fortified cereals, fortified nutritional yeast, whole eggs
Folate/Folic Acid	Prevents neural tube defects, repairs damaged cells, makes robust red and white blood cells.	Enriched grains, orange juice, legumes, spinach, broccoli, peas, strawberries
Pantothenic Acid	Production of amino acids, certain hormones, vitamins A and D, and neurotransmitters, the chemical messengers for brain cell communication.	Potatoes, broccoli, tomato products, oat cereals, whole grains, whole eggs, poultry
Niacin	Fosters normal growth in children. Releases energy from food.	Meat, milk, fish, poultry, potatoes, corn, asparagus, fortified breads and cereals, legumes

Vitamin C

Role in the body. Vitamin C is often credited with fighting off the common cold and the flu, and rightly so. Even though it cannot stop an infection, vitamin C helps the body mount a defensive response to bacteria and viruses. But vitamin

C's role in your child's health transcends that of germ buster. It's required for the production of collagen, the connective tissue that helps hold together bones, tissue, and skin; maintaining the health of cells and tissues; wound healing; and boosting the absorption of iron from food. One study in the *Journal of the American Medical Association* has noted an association between high levels of vitamin C in a child's bloodstream and lower lead levels, which may mean that vitamin C protects kids against lead poisoning, should they be exposed to this toxic mineral.

Food sources. Citrus fruits and their juices supply the most concentrated amounts of vitamin C. Here are some other good sources:

- Tomatoes and tomato juice
- Berries, particularly strawberries
- Mangoes

- Raw sweet red and green bell peppers
- Broccoli
- Kiwi

Minerals
Calcium
Role in the body. Calcium is the most abundant mineral in the body. That makes sense, since calcium is primarily responsible for shoring up bones and teeth. By the time your baby daughter reaches adulthood, her body stores of calcium will have increased by about thirty-fold; your son's by at least forty times the amount he had on board at birth.

Skeleton Crew

It's important to offer children calcium-rich foods every day. Serving them milk instead of soda and yogurt instead of cookies sets an example that should last well into their teenage years, when they will make nearly all of their own food decisions. The majority of bone growth happens during the preadolescent and adolescent years, so calcium is considered most critical from age nine and up. In fact, the suggested daily calcium requirement for nine-year-olds is 500 milligrams higher (equal to nearly 16 ounces of milk) than that of a child one year younger. When older children and teenagers skimp on calcium—as they often do—it reduces bone strength and durability, setting the stage for osteoporosis later in life. Osteoporosis is a disease characterized by brittle bones that break easily. While it's considered a condition of the aged, it has its origins in lifestyle habits that take root much earlier. For more on preventing osteoporosis, see page 219.

Calcium also regulates heartbeat and participates in muscle contraction. A calcium-rich diet beginning in infancy helps ensure that your child reaches his full potential for height and for bone thickness and strength. Calcium may also decrease the amount of lead young children absorb into their bloodstream.

In My Experience
Drink Up

I encourage my kids to drink every drop of the milk in their cereal bowls, but not just for the calcium and vitamin D milk provides. Many of the B vitamins added to breakfast cereals make their way into the milk while your child eats. Drinking the milk makes sure he gets the full benefit of the milk and cereal combination.

Food sources. Dairy products are the most concentrated calcium sources. For example, a one-, two-, or three-year-old can easily satisfy his calcium needs with just 14 ounces of most types of cow's milk or fortified soy beverages; 22 ounces a day does it for four-, five-, and six-year-old children. Legumes and vegetables contain calcium, too, but in smaller quantities. For example, your child would need more than a half cup of tofu processed with calcium to equal the calcium of 8 ounces of milk or yogurt. Breast milk and commercial formulas provide adequate calcium for infants. Here's an array of calcium-containing fare:

- Yogurt
- Cheese
- Tofu processed with calcium sulfate
- Calcium-fortified juice
- Calcium-fortified soy beverage
- Calcium-fortified breakfast cereals and grains
- Nutri-Grain cereal bars
- Kellogg's Eggo Frozen Waffles (choose Nutri-Grain Multi-Bran for the most fiber)
- Dark green leafy vegetables (excluding spinach)
- Dried figs

Covert Calcium

Here are some easy ways to sneak in calcium when kids aren't looking:

Cottage Cheese

It doesn't have as much calcium as some of its other dairy counterparts, but what it contains counts toward your child's good health.

- Stir cottage cheese into warm or cold pasta dishes, such as pasta salad.
- Blend 2 cups with 1 cup thick and chunky salsa and serve to older kids with baked tortilla chips or toasted pita bread chips.

Evaporated Milk

Evaporated milk contains twice the calcium of regular cow's milk.

- Use it when preparing mashed potatoes, macaroni and cheese, and canned cream of mushroom and tomato soups.

Powdered Milk

Talk about concentrated. One tablespoon of powdered milk contains as much calcium as a third of a cup of fluid milk.

- Add a tablespoon of powdered milk to your child's hot cocoa (but make sure it's tepid, not hot!) or to a blended fruit smoothie.
- Thicken casseroles with powdered milk.

Iron

Role in the body. Iron helps carry oxygen to all the cells in the body. It plays a particularly vital role in brain development and function by promoting communication among nerve cells and by ensuring the quality of the central nervous system. For more on iron and brain function, see page 59.

What your baby eats during the first year of life determines his risk for iron deficiency later on. Most likely, your son was born with all the iron he needs for up to six months, but he will quickly use up his stored iron to fuel growth.

Food sources. Breast milk and iron-fortified formulas are excellent iron sources for baby. Breast milk actually contains much less iron than commercial infant formulas, but the iron is well absorbed by the body, making it a much better iron source than low-iron formulas or cow's milk. If you bottle-feed your baby, you should opt for iron-fortified infant formulas, as there is no scientific evidence that says parents should do otherwise. In fact, choosing low-iron commercial formulas to feed your healthy baby poses a risk for iron deficiency.

Iron comes in two forms: heme and nonheme. Heme iron is best absorbed by the body. It's found in varying amounts in animal foods. Nonheme iron is the only type of iron in plant foods. Most processed grains also contain added nonheme iron.

You can find heme iron in:

- Clams
- Oysters
- Beef and other meats (including jarred meats for baby)
- Poultry
- Pork
- Egg yolk

Good sources for nonheme iron include:

- Iron-fortified infant cereal
- Iron-fortified infant formula
- Spinach
- Potatoes
- Raisins
- Legumes
- Fortified bread, cereal, rice, pasta, and other grains

Coming Up Short

In spite of the wide array of iron-rich foods available, iron deficiency is the most common nutritional shortfall among American children. Why? Kids under the age of three are at risk because they grow so quickly. When a child's dietary intake of iron does not match his needs, the result is iron deficiency. More often than not, a faulty diet is to blame, although there are other reasons for low body-iron stores. Premature babies, infants who did not grow properly during pregnancy, and children born to moms with diabetes are at greater risk for an iron deficiency because of their lower-than-normal iron reserves at birth. If your baby was premature or weighed less than 5.5 pounds at delivery, she is more likely to become iron deficient by two to three months. That's because underweight babies grow more rapidly than full-term babies after birth, using up their already-limited iron stores that much faster.

The most notable consequence of iron deficiency is anemia (anemia can be caused by a number of other factors, too). But your child doesn't have to be diagnosed with anemia to suffer from iron deficiency. Because of its many vital functions in brain growth and overall development, a lack of iron in infants and young children may have long-term repercussions. Iron deficiency has negative effects on a child's capacity for learning, possibly by reducing his attention span and his responsiveness to his surroundings. Some experts say that these early cognitive losses may not be reversible, even when iron deficiency is discovered and corrected through supplementation and other dietary improvements.

Another little-known result of iron deficiency concerns the toxic mineral lead. Kids with low body-iron reserves are more likely to absorb lead from their intestinal tract. The combination of iron deficiency and increased blood lead levels causes permanent neurological and developmental problems.

Pumping Iron

Nonheme iron, the type found primarily in plant foods, is not well absorbed by the body. Yet, studies show it's an important iron source for children, especially for those who don't eat meat or who completely avoid animal foods. You can boost the body's nonheme iron uptake in two ways: by serving foods rich in nonheme iron along with a source of vitamin C, and by combining them with foods packed with heme iron, such as beef, pork, and poultry. For instance, serve kids juice high in vitamin C along with their iron-fortified breakfast cereal or with toast made from fortified bread. (However, calcium-fortified juice, a vitamin C source, decreases iron absorption somewhat.) The iron in a fortified bun gets a boost from the heme iron in the burger; adding sliced tomato and strawberries to the meal further increases the body's nonheme iron absorption.

Sodium

Role in the body. You may have a love-hate relationship with sodium: You love it because it adds flavor to foods, but you despise it because of its supposed ill effects. Sodium gets little respect for its true functions, however. It's necessary for proper fluid balance; muscle contraction; nerve conduction; and the transport of nutrients into, and wastes out of, your child's cells.

When it comes to sodium, there's no question your healthy child will get enough. That's because every food contains some sodium. The issue with sodium is how much is too much. We know that in certain salt-sensitive adults, excessive sodium intake may actually cause high blood pressure, but it's uncertain what a high intake does to kids, and if any negative health effects are lasting. When a child has high blood pressure, overweight may be to blame rather than sodium. Even in children as young as two, carrying around extra pounds has been associated with elevated blood pressure readings. Chronically high blood pressure is a risk factor for heart disease and stroke in adults.

Food sources. Mother Nature made sure sodium is present in every food, but processed foods take the cake for sodium content. Experts say that most of the sodium in the American diet comes from salt (which is actually sodium and chloride bound together) added during processing and manufacturing. That means convenience foods, including such kid-favorites as frozen potato puffs, bologna, and canned spaghetti contribute most of the sodium to a child's diet. Here are some other sodium-filled foods:

- Boxed macaroni and cheese
- Canned soups and vegetables
- Cold cuts
- Hot dogs
- Lunchables
- Snack chips

In My Experience
Vitamin and Mineral Supplements Provide Security

"Do you give your kids vitamins?" That's a question parents ask me again and again. The answer is an unqualified yes. And here's why.

Children should get the bulk of nutrients from foods, and as a dietitian, this is the route I prefer. But I am a realist. Despite having a dietitian for a mother, my kids do not eat exemplary diets, and I bet your child doesn't, either.

I do serve my kids healthy foods (well, OK, not *all* the time), but truth be told, they are not much for the variety I encourage, nor do they love the idea of eating five servings of fruits and vegetables every day. None of my three daughters eats much beef or seafood, even though my husband and I regularly offer it to them in small quantities. Each child seems to go through eating jags that can last for weeks, when she refuses the foods that she typically loves. Their erratic eating habits make for a shortfall of nutrients during any given week. So, in order to cover the bases, I give my two oldest daughters a daily chewable multivitamin/multimineral pill that includes iron and zinc—two nutrients that often go missing when a child doesn't eat meat with regularity; the youngest gets half of a chewable multivitamin. I choose supplements that provide no more than about 100 percent of the Daily Value (DV) for the nutrients listed on the label.

Dietary supplements provide parents with a certain sense of security, and children get a safety net should their diets fall short. But supplements are just what their name implies. They are not substitutes for a healthy diet. While concentrated vitamin and mineral liquids and pills can fill nutrient gaps, they cannot supply the calories, carbohydrate, fat, protein, fiber, or calcium a growing child needs. There is no reason to give a healthy child large doses of any nutrient unless your pediatrician advises it.

Zinc

Role in the body. You may not think too often about zinc, even though it's important enough to be present in every organ, tissue, and bodily fluid and secretion. It's remarkable that zinc does not garner more attention, since it's crucial for cell growth (including brain tissue) and repair, energy production, insulin production, and a healthy immune system. It's common for kids to consume less than the recommended amount of zinc, even when they are otherwise well nourished.

Food sources. With the exception of oysters, beef packs the most zinc. Plant foods supply zinc, too, but the body doesn't absorb it as well as the zinc in animal products. Some plant foods such as whole grains, legumes, and soy products contain phytates, which block zinc absorption to some degree. Strict vegetarians may have difficulty getting the zinc they need from diet alone. Here are some additional zinc-rich foods:

- Fortified breakfast cereals
- Lamb
- Legumes (including peas)
- Milk
- Pork
- Poultry, particularly dark meat
- Wheat germ cereal
- Yogurt (plain contains the most)

Fluoride

Role in the body. Dental experts say that fluoride is to thank in large part for the decline in childhood cavities in developed countries, including the United States. Studies show that the earlier in life your youngster is exposed to fluoride, the greater the chance for reducing cavities in her primary and permanent teeth. Fluoride protects your child's teeth throughout life, too.

Fluoride works in two ways to defend teeth. Before your child ever cuts a tooth, fluoride is there behind the scenes, shoring up enamel, the tooth's protective outer surface. Stronger enamel is more resistant to cavity-causing acid produced by the bacteria that live in the mouth. After teeth appear, fluoride lowers the germs' acid production, further reducing cavity risk.

Fluoride also plays a role in bone health. It shows promise for prompting the body to form new bone tissue. And fluoride has been used as a drug to combat osteoporosis, a disease that leaves bones susceptible to fracture.

Food sources. Babies and youngsters can most easily reap the benefits of fluoride by drinking from a municipal water supply that contains added fluoride. The majority of municipal water is fluoridated, but if you have any doubt, ask your city or town's water department if the tap water supplies fluoride. Certain kid-appropriate beverages, including decaffeinated tea, are particularly rich in fluoride, and are even higher when prepared with fluoridated water. Formula-fed infants may receive adequate fluoride when the commercial powdered or liquid-concentrate infant formula they drink is made with fluoridated water. Your baby may not get enough fluoride if you use bottled water to prepare infant formula, however. If you prefer bottled water over tap, call the company to find out how much fluoride is in the water your baby drinks, then ask your pediatrician if the amount is adequate. Breastfed babies don't require a fluoride supplement for the first six months of life but may need one after that if they don't drink fluoridated water.

Once your daughter starts brushing her teeth, fluoridated toothpaste becomes a major nonfood fluoride source. Too much fluoride early in life can cause mottling of the teeth, which is more of a cosmetic flaw than anything. In other words, it may look bad, but it probably won't affect the strength of the teeth. For more information on the role of fluoride and other nutrients in cavity prevention, see page 211.

"FIGHT-O" CHEMICALS: NATURE'S WEAPONRY

With names like *isoflavenoids*, *tangeretin*, *nobiletin*, and *beta-cryptoxanthin*, it's no wonder that you might be put off by phytochemicals. Just the word *phytochemical* can intimidate, but it shouldn't. Put simply, phytochemicals are the substances present in plant foods, including fruits, vegetables, legumes, and grains. When it comes to "phytos," nothing could be more natural, or good for you.

Neither vitamins nor minerals, the thousands of phytochemicals found in plant foods are garnering increasing attention for their role in good health. Scientists suspect that phytochemicals help fight off the cancer, cataracts, and heart disease that could be in your child's future. In addition, the likes of lycopene, lutein, and limonene provide plants with their color, aroma, and flavor. What's more, they boost a plant's natural self-defense system, helping it to resist the effects of extreme weather conditions and harsh sunlight.

How do phytochemicals work in humans? Some phytos perform as antioxidants, thwarting cell damage that could be the beginnings of disease. Other phytos act to stimulate anticancer enzymes, and still others whisk potential cancer-causing agents out of the body.

Feeding kids a variety of plant foods is the best way to load them up with an arsenal of disease-fighting phytos. As long as it's fresh or lightly processed, experts say that every fruit, vegetable, nut, legume, and grain has something to offer by way of phytochemicals. For example, a single orange supplies more than 170 different beneficial substances with a wide array of health benefits. Phytochemical supplements have not been proven to have the same health effects as their naturally occurring counterparts.

Children and Herbs: Not a Good Mix

Botanicals are big business. An estimated 60 million Americans have tried botanical supplements such as feverfew (to prevent migraines), echinacea (to prevent cold symptoms), ginger (for nausea), and St. John's wort (to boost mood). No doubt, so have many children. And that raises a red flag.

Sure, herbal remedies seem safe enough. After all, botanical products are made from plants, right? But when you take herbs to feel better; to keep from getting a cold or flu; or to "cure" ear infections, bronchitis, asthma, and Attention Deficit Hyperactivity Disorder, they take on druglike qualities.

Problem is, botanicals are not regulated as drugs in this country. The FDA classifies them as dietary supplements, and as such, botanicals are immune to the tough testing for safety and effectiveness that over-the-counter and prescription medications are subjected to. That means that anyone can produce dietary supplements and sell them without the approval of the FDA and without the years of rigorous testing that medications must have before they are considered safe for consumers' use. Lax regulation means there's no guarantee that consumers get the botanical they pay for, or that the product contains enough of the active ingredients to make a difference.

That's not to say that botanicals, including herbal remedies such as ginkgo, valerian, and saw palmetto, are without scientific merit. Certain botanicals have been studied extensively, mostly in Europe. So what's the problem with botanical remedies? Many have not been adequately investigated, calling into question their safety and efficacy. More to the point: The effects of most botanicals on children are unknown. Experts do know this: Children lack the liver enzymes to metabolize many medications, including botanicals. The bottom line is never treat a child with a botanical remedy without telling your pediatrician first. Many plant products can cause allergic reactions, and some interfere with other medication your child may be taking.

FLUID

Role in the body. Fluid is often overlooked as a nutrient. Fluid qualifies as an essential part of the diet, since you must get water from outside sources to survive. In fact, water may be thought of as the most vital of nutrients, if there is such as thing. After all, every life-giving bodily process takes place in a watery environment. Without water, your child's body wouldn't be able to regulate its internal temperature; transport nutrients to cells and waste products away from them; moisten the digestive tract; cushion and protect tissues, organs, and joints from injury; and produce much-needed energy.

Water Works

How much water for your child? Experts link water needs to calorie intake when making suggestions for fluid. Here are some general guidelines based on recommended calories.

Age	Recommended Daily Fluid Intake (ounces)
Birth to 6 months*	32
6 to 12 months	42
1 to 3 years	64
4 to 6 years	88

*Infants do not need water in addition to formula or breast milk.

You need fluid every day to function. That's because the body loses water, largely through sweating, urinating, and breathing. Water is necessary to make the urine that rids the body of waste products from metabolism. Sweating is the way the body gives off heat generated by everyday bodily processes and physical activity. That's critical, since your internal core temperature must hover around 98.6°F for optimum health. Water, in the form of vapor, also evaporates from the respiratory tract in breathing.

Do babies need water? Generally speaking, they do not because breast milk and formula contain adequate fluid. Infants who nurse or take infant formula only do not generally require extra water, unless the weather is hot. In fact, too much water can be dangerous to babies, according to the AAP. Excessive water consumption in infants can cause the condition known as water intoxication. Water intoxication is when the body cannot rid itself of the water it has on board; the condition can be life threatening. The AAP warns that giving a lot of extra water to babies who are not eating solid foods may mean that they won't drink adequate amounts of breast milk or formula. In fact, water intoxication is more likely to occur in babies fed only formula or breast milk and less likely in those who eat table foods, too. When it seems that your child just can't get enough fluid and he or she urinates too often, notify your pediatrician. The combination of excessive thirst and urination may be a sign of diabetes.

Water: Tap or Bottled?

Labels picturing pristine mountain tops or springs may lead you to believe that bottled water is better for your family, but is it? Perhaps. Depending on your water supply, bottled water may be a healthier choice. Here's what to consider when deciding between bottled water and water from a municipal supply.

- **Lead.** Public drinking water is usually lead-free as it leaves treatment plants. Problems arise when lead leaches into water from the lead pipes and solder in dwellings. By contrast, bottled water typically contains no lead.
- **Fluoride**. With the exception of a few brands, bottled water lacks adequate fluoride for developing teeth. Make sure your pediatrician and dentist know if you are using bottled water to make infant formula or if bottled water is your child's sole source of water. Baby may need a fluoride supplement.
- **Chlorine.** Municipalities use chlorine to kill germs in their water supplies. Chlorine can leave an undesirable aftertaste. Even worse, it can be a health hazard. When chlorine meets up with naturally occurring matter such as leaves, it combines with them to form compounds called disinfection byproducts (DBP). According to the EPA, the agency that determines drinking water standards, long-term consumption of water with DBP levels that exceed safe levels increases the risk of certain cancers. Preliminary data suggest chlorinated water may cause miscarriage, too. According to the International Bottled Water Association, bottlers eschew chlorine for other ways to disinfect water, including ozone and ultraviolet light. Millions of Americans drink water from private wells. The EPA does not oversee private drinking sources, but the organization provides excellent tips for keeping them safe at *www.epa.gov/safewater.*
- **Quality and price.** Twenty-five percent of the bottled water we drink is actually from community or municipal water sources. You may not want to pay a premium for tap water, so check the label for the source. Choose brands bottled by companies who are members of the International Bottled Water Association to ensure higher water quality.

Fluid sources. Water is the best fluid source because it is most rapidly absorbed into the bloodstream from the digestive tract. Even so, other beverages such as milk and juice help satisfy a child's fluid needs, too. Lettuce, tomatoes, broccoli, oranges, apricots, and apples are among the foods highest in water content; the fattiest foods contribute the least water to the diet. Encouraging children to eat the recommended five servings of fruits and vegetables a day goes a long way toward helping them meet their fluid requirements.

Dodging Dehydration

Children, particularly infants, are prone to dehydration. For starters, smaller stature makes for quicker water loss in youngsters. Younger kids also have more skin surface in relation to their body weight, which provides greater opportunity for fluid loss through sweating. In addition, little tikes have more trouble conserving water than older people because their kidneys are not as effective at keeping water on board.

As your child matures and moves around more, he requires additional fluid before, during, and after play, especially when it's hot and humid outside and when it's very cold (weather extremes use up more water for proper body temperature regulation). Prolonged vomiting or diarrhea (or both) increases fluid loss and puts kids at particular risk for dehydration. When children, particularly infants, have large, frequent, watery stools, consult your pediatrician about the need for a rehydrating solution. During times of intestinal illness, plain water is not always the best option because children lose important nutrients called electrolytes that cannot be replenished with plain water. Electrolytes are vital to maintaining the body's chemical balance.

Depending on his age, your child cannot always tell you when he needs fluid. But even if he can talk about his thirst, it's not wise to wait until he asks for a beverage to encourage fluid intake. That's because thirst actually signals dehydration. Additional symptoms of dehydration include dry mouth, flushed skin, fatigue, headache, lethargy, fever, increased breathing rate and pulse, dizziness, increased weakness, and labored breathing. The color and amount of urine your child produces is telling, too. Small quantities of deeply colored urine mean your son is not meeting his fluid needs. Urine is slightly darker in the morning in older children. That's because they have typically gone without peeing for eight hours, so urine is more concentrated. Concentrated urine is darker.

For the most part, getting your child to drink is the best way to dodge dehydration. Kids who are playing or participating in an organized sport should be encouraged to sip three to four ounces of fluid every fifteen minutes or so. If they find water boring, diluted fruit juices may be more acceptable to them. Don't leave home without fluid. When you are out and about, bring along water in kid-friendly containers, small juice boxes, or take milk in a cooler or thermos.

Cut the Caffeine

Caffeine causes water loss from the body, never mind the fact that it can make kids bonkers and interfere with their sleep. As little as 200 milligrams of caffeine at a time can cause nervousness and anxiety in adults who don't usually consume caffeine. It takes much less caffeine to produce the same effects in kids.

You know that caffeine is not good for children, but it's getting harder to figure out which foods contain caffeine, because it's not listed on food labels. Coffee, colas, and tea are the obvious sources, but manufacturers add caffeine to other foods, including orange soda and water. Then there are coffee-flavored foods to consider.

The Center for Science in the Public Interest (CSPI) wants to make it easier for parents and others to keep track of caffeine intake. The organization has asked the FDA to require manufacturers to list a product's precise caffeine content. While the agency is still considering the request, study this list to help keep your child caffeine free.

Caffeine Amounts

Food	Caffeine (milligrams)	Food	Caffeine (milligrams)
Brewed coffee, 8 ounces	135	Diet Coke, 12 ounces	47
Java Water, 8 ounces	63	Coca-Cola, 12 ounces	45
Josta soda, 12 ounces	58	Dannon Coffee Yogurt,	
Mountain Dew, 12 ounces	55	8 ounces	45
Surge, 12 ounces	51	Ben & Jerry's No Fat Coffee	
Tea, steeped from leaf		Fudge Frozen Yogurt,	
or a tea bag, 8 ounces	50	½ cup	43
Krank20, 8 ounces	50	Sunkist Orange Soda,	
Snapple Iced Tea,		12 ounces	40
all varieties, 16 ounces	48	Pepsi Cola, 12 ounces	37

(continued)

Caffeine Amounts *(continued)*

Food	Caffeine (milligrams)	Food	Caffeine (milligrams)
Hershey's Special Dark		7-UP, 12 ounces	0
Chocolate Bar, 1.5 ounces	31	Minute Maid Orange Soda,	
Häagen-Dazs Coffee Ice		12 ounces	0
Cream, ½ cup	29	Mug Root Beer, 12 ounces	0
Barq's Root Beer, 12 ounces	23	Sprite or Diet Sprite,	
Hershey Bar, 1.5 ounces	10	12 ounces	0
Yoplait Cafe au Lait Yogurt,		Stonyfield Farm Mocha Latte	
6 ounces	5	Yogurt, 6 ounces	0

Judging Juice

Parents tend to think of fruit juice as a healthy, kid-friendly beverage, almost as good for you as milk and much better than soda. Just six ounces of fruit juice counts as one of the recommended five or more daily servings from the fruit group of the Food Guide Pyramid. And 100 percent fruit juice contains vitamins, minerals, and disease-fighting phytochemicals. When juice producers add extra nutrients, juice looks even better to parents and nutritionists: Orange juice fortified with calcium and extra vitamin C is a great way for children to consume more nutrients without drinking a lot of low-fiber, high-calorie beverages.

It may come from fruit, but when it comes to juice, you can have too much of a good thing. According to a study published in *Pediatrics,* children between the ages of two and five who drink at least 12 ounces of fruit juice daily are shorter and heavier than those who drink less. Why? Perhaps it's because juice is a high-calorie beverage that's appealing to kids because of its sweetness, making it easy for them to load up on extra calories. As for short stature, excessive juice drinking can displace milk from your child's diet. Milk contains calcium and vitamin D that help bones grow in length and thickness.

Do kids need juice? Technically speaking, no. With the exception of added calcium, children can get the same nutrients by eating fruit, which provides the fiber that juice does not. Is there anything wrong with juice drinking? No, as long as you limit your child's consumption and choose wisely. Here are some juicy tips.

(continued)

- Limit juice intake to 6 ounces a day in children six and under.
- Purchase only 100 percent fruit juice products for the biggest nutritional bang for the buck.
- Avoid concoctions whose names contain the following: *beverage, cocktail, drink, blend,* or *-ade* (like *lemonade*). These are mixtures that contain some juice combined with water and sweeteners. Some brands have all-juice products and products with very little juice, so read the label—it must state the juice content.
- Never serve your child juice from a baby bottle. If he is old enough to drink juice, then he should be sipping it from a cup, covered or not, depending on his skills. Allowing babies and toddlers to suck on a juice bottle at will encourages cavities since it supplies a steady stream of carbohydrate that can pool around teeth and lead to holes in tooth enamel.
- Opt for diluted fortified juice such as calcium-added cranberry or orange juice, or apple juice with vitamin C. Fortified mixtures of high fructose corn syrup (sugar), water, and juice don't provide the full benefits of 100 percent juice products.

Fluid Fun

Fluid is more than water. In fact, any food that is liquid at room temperature, such as ice cream and frozen pops, counts toward a child's fluid needs. When kids complain that plain water is a bore, try these tactics to foster fluid intake.

Freeze it. Blenderize a combination of your favorite berries. Partially freeze in ice cube trays or in small paper cups. Have kids eat with a spoon.

Zing it. Keep a pitcher of ice-cold water and lemon, lime, or orange slices on hand in the refrigerator.

Mix it. Combine club soda or seltzer water with a splash of 100 percent fruit juice.

Pop it. Freeze diluted 100 percent fruit juice in ice-pop molds.

Sip it. Prepare a smoothie by mixing eight ounces of milk, a banana, and one or two ice cubes. Serve to kids with a straw.

PYRAMID POWER

You may have grown up with the four food groups, but your children will use a different guide for healthy eating: the United States Department of Agriculture's (USDA) Food Guide Pyramid. With its five food groups, the pyramid stresses the importance of plant foods as the basis of a healthy diet.

The USDA's Food Guide for Young Children is an adaptation of the original Food Guide Pyramid and is designed specifically for children ages two to six. While the kid-friendly version of the Food Guide Pyramid emphasizes choosing a variety of foods, it differs from the original in several ways, including recognizing that some fats are necessary for early growth and development, going with shorter food group names and more succinct recommendations for servings from each group, including foods commonly eaten by kids, and emphasizing physical activity as part of a healthy lifestyle. Both pyramids provide a tool for meal planning for kids, making healthy eating easier on parents and other caregivers.

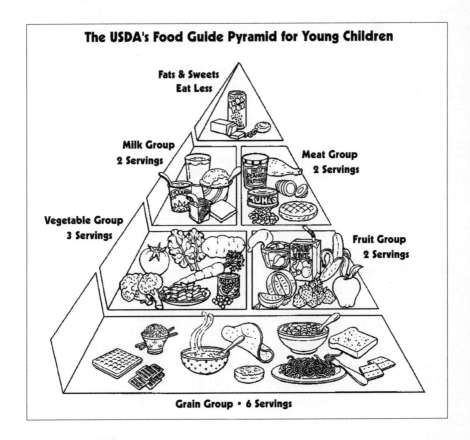

The USDA's Food Guide Pyramid for Young Children

Fats & Sweets
Eat Less

Milk Group
2 Servings

Meat Group
2 Servings

Vegetable Group
3 Servings

Fruit Group
2 Servings

Grain Group • 6 Servings

The Pyramid Plan

With the exception of the tip of the pyramid, which houses highly caloric, low-nutrient fats and sweets, the relative size of the food groups does not dictate their importance. Each is crucial to a child's growth and development. The Milk Group and the Meat Group may occupy less space on the pyramid graphic than the Grain Group, but that doesn't diminish their role in a healthy diet: the Grain Group is bigger because foods from that category should dominate a youngster's eating plan. Many kids go through periods of refusing to eat foods from one or more of the food groups. This is not typically a problem unless it is prolonged. When it goes on for weeks or months with no end in sight, consult a registered dietitian. She can help you compensate for missing nutrients by recommending suitable substitutes for the food your little one avoids.

Size Matters

Portion size is paramount to healthy eating. While nearly all foods fit into a diet that fosters peak growth and development, too little food from one group or too much from another wreaks havoc with the dietary balance that nutritionists recommend.

Now that you know the number of servings to offer your child, your next question probably concerns serving size. That's where the following lists come in. They explain how much food from each of the five groups in the Food Guide Pyramid constitutes a kid-size portion. Portions are key to planning nutritious meals and snacks.

Yet, there is a caveat. Portion sizes and number of servings from the Food Guide Pyramid are guidelines for good eating, not mandates. Why? A child's appetite can vary widely, given all of the rapid changes taking place in her body, including teething and getting taller. Physical activity also affects how much a child consumes. That's why there will be times when your daughter eats the recommended amounts as explained here, and times when she eats more food. Also, keep in mind that the Food Guide Pyramid for Young Children is meant for two- to six-year-olds and that the youngest kids in this category will eat less than older children.

Don't feel pressured by the prescribed amounts, particularly when offering new foods. Introduce very small portions of new foods, rather than the full portion described in the food lists. It's OK to start small (about a tablespoon of food per year of age) and work your way up as your child gradually incorporates different foods into her eating plan. For example, serve up a small cooked broccoli floret instead of the full kid-size serving of two broccoli spears.

Here's how the lists work together with the pyramid diagram. The portion sizes below are actually intended for children ages four and above. Serve two- and three-year-olds about two-thirds of the following kid-friendly portions and count it as a serving. The Milk Group is the exception to this rule. Children two through six need at least two full servings (as listed) a day from the Milk Group, so don't decrease daily dairy portions.

Grain Group (6 servings per day)

Key nutrients: Carbohydrate, fiber (especially in whole grains), B vitamins such as the folic acid found in enriched grains, and iron in fortified products.

Offer whole grain or enriched grain choices more often.

A serving is:

- ½ cup cooked grain such as rice, pasta, grits, or oatmeal
- 1 ounce ready-to-eat cereal, preferably whole grain
- 5–6 whole grain crackers
- 3 cups popped popcorn*
- 1 slice bread (1 ounce)
- ½ English muffin or bagel (1 ounce)
- 2 taco shells*
- 1 7-inch corn or flour tortilla
- ½ hamburger or hot dog bun
- 1 small roll (1 ounce)
- 1 4-inch pita bread
- 1 4-inch pancake or waffle
- 9 3-ring pretzels*

Selections with more added fat and sugar:

- 1 small biscuit or muffin
- 1 small piece cornbread
- ½ medium doughnut
- 9 animal crackers
- 4 small cookies

*Avoid in children under the age of four because of choking hazard.

Vegetable Group (2 servings per day)

Key nutrients: Carbohydrate, fiber, folate (the naturally occurring form of folic acid), disease-fighting phytochemicals, vitamins C and E.

A serving is:

- ½ cup cooked green leafy vegetables such as spinach and collard greens
- 1 cup leafy raw vegetables such as salad greens
- 2 cooked broccoli spears
- 1½ carrots, cooked
- 7–8 raw carrot or celery sticks (3 inches long)*
- ½ cup cooked winter squash

- 1 medium ear of corn*
- ½ cup green peas*
- ½ cup lima beans
- 1 medium plantain
- ⅓ medium cucumber, peeled
- 9 raw snow or sugar snap pea pods
- ½ cup cooked green beans
- 4 medium brussels sprouts
- 6 slices raw summer squash
- ½ cup cooked cabbage
- ½ cup tomato or spaghetti sauce
- ¾ cup (6 ounces) vegetable juice
- 1 cup vegetable soup
- 1 medium tomato
- 5 cherry tomatoes*

Choices that also double as meat alternates because of their high protein content:
- ½ cup cooked legumes such as black, kidney, and garbanzo beans
- ½ cup cooked lentils
- 1 cup bean soup
- ½ cup cooked split peas

Choices that are higher in fat:
- 10 French fries
- ½ cup potato salad
- ½ cup coleslaw

*Avoid in children under the age of four because of choking hazard.

Fruit Group (2 servings per day)
Key nutrients: Carbohydrate, fiber, folate (the naturally occurring form of folic acid), disease-fighting phytochemicals, vitamin C.

A serving is:
- ½ cup berries or 7 medium strawberries
- ¼ medium cantaloupe
- ¾ cup (6 ounces) 100 percent fruit juice
- ½ grapefruit
- ⅛ honeydew melon
- 1 large kiwi

- 1 medium orange, tangerine, apple, banana, peach, or nectarine
- 2 medium apricots
- ½ cup watermelon, cubed
- 11 cherries*
- ¼ cup dried fruit*
- ½ cup applesauce, preferably unsweetened
- 2½ pineapple slices
- 12 grapes*
- ½ medium mango
- ¼ medium papaya
- 1 small pear
- ½ cup fresh, canned, or cooked fruit, cut up

*Avoid in children under the age of four because of choking hazard.

Milk Group (All ages require at least 2 servings per day)

Key nutrients: Carbohydrate, protein, fat, B vitamins, calcium and other bone-building minerals, vitamin D (in milk).

A serving is:
- 8 ounces milk (any type)
- 8 ounces calcium-fortified soy beverage
- 1 cup yogurt (8 ounces)
- 1½ ounces natural cheese such as cheddar or Swiss
- 2 ounces processed cheese such as American
- 1 string cheese (1 ounce)
- 2 cups cottage cheese
- 1½ cups ice cream
- 1 cup frozen yogurt
- 1 cup pudding

Meat Group

Key nutrients: Protein, fat (especially in higher fat cuts of fresh meat and processed varieties, fattier fish such as salmon, nuts and nut butters, tofu), iron, zinc, fiber (legumes), B vitamins, and choline (in eggs and beef).

The Meat Group is different from the rest but no harder to figure out. Two- and three-year-olds should eat a total of about 3½ ounces (a little bit bigger than a deck of cards) of cooked lean meat, poultry, or seafood or the equivalent every day; four-, five-, and six-year-olds need about 5 ounces daily.

Count the following meat equivalents as 1 ounce of meat:
- 1 whole egg
- 2 tablespoons peanut butter*
- 1½ frankfurters (2 ounces total)**
- 2 slices luncheon meat (2 ounces)**
- ¼ cup drained canned salmon or tuna
- ½ cup cooked kidney beans or other legumes
- ½ cup tofu
- 1 soy burger patty

*Avoid in children under the age of four because of choking hazard.

**High-fat, high-sodium choices that should be the exception rather than the rule in menu planning for your youngster.

Fats and Sweets

The small size of this group says it all, loud and clear: Use fats and sugar sparingly. Easier said than done, I admit. The choices belonging to this category, including candy and sugary soft drinks, can be the bane of a parent's existence. Kids crave them, and even when parents give in, kids will complain about their limited portions. Moderation is the key to managing foods that contain high concentrations of sugar and fat. You don't have to severely restrict the likes of butter, margarine, and cooking oil. On the other hand, don't go overboard on fatty cookies and pastries, which technically fall into the Grain Group but which fit better into the Fats and Sweets Group, given their negligible nutritional worth.

Sample Menu: Ages Two Through Six

With all the choices the Food Guide Pyramid for Young Children provides, menu planning possibilities are endless. This sample one-day menu is simply a suggestion for youngsters. Remember to decrease portions by about a third for two- and three-year-olds, with the exception of the Milk Group servings.

Breakfast
- 1 medium banana (1 Fruit)
- 2 ounces fortified cereal (2 Grain)
- 8 ounces milk (1 Milk)

Snack
- 5 whole grain crackers (1 Grain)
- 1½ ounces hard cheese such as cheddar (½ Milk)

Lunch
- 2 ounces turkey or chicken (2 Meat)
- 1 teaspoon mayonnaise (Fats and Sweets)
- 2 slices whole grain bread (2 Grains)
- 4 ounces milk (½ Milk)

Snack
- 7–8 3-inch-long raw carrot sticks. Serve cooked carrots to kids under four. (1 Vegetable)
- 1 tablespoon peanut butter for dipping (½ Meat)
- 6 ounces calcium-fortified 100 percent fruit juice (1 Fruit)

Dinner
- Meat, poultry, or fish, 2 ounces, cooked (2 Meat)
- 2 cooked broccoli spears (1 Vegetable)
- 1 medium roll or biscuit (1 Grain)
- 1 teaspoon butter or margarine (Fats and Sweets)
- 4 ounces milk (½ Milk)

Snack
- 1 medium piece of fruit (1 Fruit)

If You Serve It, They Will Eat

The bigger the portion, the more kids consume, especially older preschoolers. That's according to a study in the *Journal of the American Dietetic Association.* Researchers studying groups of three- and five-year-olds found that the older children polished off the food placed in front of them regardless of portion size, while their younger counterparts appeared to stop eating when full. The lesson: Start with small portions. If your child is still hungry, serve more.

Infants and Toddlers: How Much Food Is Enough?

Feeding infants and very young toddlers can be tough. Once your child begins solid foods, it's difficult to determine how much to serve. And just when you've established a feeding "routine," it changes yet again.

The Food Guide Pyramid for Young Children is useful for children over the age of two, but if your child is not there yet, what should guide you in the meantime?

Although babies may begin solid foods at four months, six months is more like it. As your little tike begins eating more new foods and drinking less breast milk or formula, his intake will be erratic. That's perfectly normal. By the time he is a year old, he will probably be feeding himself finger foods and could be drinking from a covered cup. Remember, while there are developmental milestones children should reach by a certain age, each child is unique, so don't worry if your baby hasn't mastered using a fork or spoon by eighteen months, even if your friend's or neighbor's baby has.

Around your son's first birthday, he can begin making the transition from breast milk or infant formula to whole milk. You may choose to nurse for longer than a year. That's fine, but there is really no need for a baby to drink formula past this point as long as he is eating well. (Babies with milk allergies may be the exception.) In fact, serving baby too much formula can promote a reliance on it for calories and detract from solid foods. This is also the time when baby can begin weaning himself from a bottle. See Chapter 6 for ways to feed your one-year-old.

Chapter 3

Food Power: More Than an Apple a Day

My job as a parent is to provide my kids with the best possible start, and that means serving them the most nutritious foods.

—*Janice, mother of two girls*

When mom told you to finish your vegetables and to drink all of your milk, she knew she was doing a good thing, but she probably didn't know all the reasons why. There's no question good nutrition fosters peak physical and intellectual potential. Scientific studies have come to prove what mom knew intuitively all along: A healthy diet during childhood reduces the risk of developing chronic conditions, including osteoporosis, heart disease, and cancer, later in life.

PUT NUTRITION TO WORK

No single nutrient, food, or food group is the ticket to wellness, which is one of the reasons nutrition experts recommend eating a variety of foods. Nutrients work together to promote health, sometimes within single foods; in whole meals; and in an entire diet. The dynamic duo of calcium and vitamin D in milk is a case in point. Milk is a concentrated calcium source, and it is the primary dairy food fortified with vitamin D. (Some yogurt may contain added vitamin D.) Vitamin D boosts calcium absorption, helping this much-needed mineral make its way into bones to provide strength. Another example of nutrient teamwork occurs in enriched grains. Nutrient-packed grains such as bread and breakfast cereal contain carbohydrate as well as B vitamins. That's beneficial because you need B vitamins to free up the calories carbohydrate contains so that your body can make use of the energy.

Arguably, all foods and nutrients are critical for a growing child, but here are some standouts that should not be missed.

Fatty Fuel

You may be avoiding fat in the name of reducing your waistline or in the hopes of heading off heart disease. But kids need this concentrated calorie source to support rapid growth and to promote peak mental acumen.

The omega-3 fats found primarily in seafood are especially worthy of mention, since they play a vital role in brain development and proper visual development during gestation and the first two years of life. These same fats are good for the whole family. Omega-3s may protect adults against heart disease, stroke, rheumatoid arthritis, high blood pressure, and cancer, while boosting immune function, preserving vision, and fighting off depression, according to preliminary research.

Produce Power

Population studies suggest that people who eat the most fruits and vegetables enjoy a greatly reduced risk of developing cancers of the lung, cervix, esophagus, stomach, colon, pancreas, breast, and prostate, as well as a lower likelihood of developing heart disease. In addition, the phytochemicals in fruits, vegetables, and grains may protect eyesight, prevent heart disease, and thwart urinary tract infections.

Produce builds bones, too. Green leafy vegetables such as broccoli, lettuce, cabbage, and kale contain vitamin K, a nutrient that is vital to bone tissue formation through its role in producing a protein necessary for a sturdy skeleton. Research conducted at the Harvard School of Public Health found that midlife women who consumed nearly double the Recommended Dietary Allowance (RDA) for vitamin K every day from food had the lowest rate of hip fractures. While the subjects of this study were adults, there's little reason to doubt that produce bolsters a child's bones, too.

In addition, fruits and vegetables help to keep blood pressure in check. The Dietary Approaches to Stop Hypertension (DASH) study found that eating a low-fat diet packed with produce, whole grain products, and two to three servings of high-calcium, low-fat dairy products lowered blood pressure in adults as successfully as prescription medication. No one can pinpoint the exact reason why the DASH diet is effective, but researchers say that the combination of foods may be what holds down blood pressure readings.

No dietary supplement has yet harnessed the power of the thousands of different phytochemicals packed in plant foods, so kids should eat fruits and vegetables every day as part of a balanced diet. Everyone benefits from phytochemicals by following the eating regimen suggested by the USDA Food Guide Pyramid. The pyramid (see page 43) promotes a diet based on grains, breads, cereal, pasta, and at least five daily servings of fruits and vegetables. For more information about kid-size produce portions and how to make eating fruits and vegetables more fun, see page 130.

A Dose of Dairy

Calcium is needed for strong teeth and bones, to curb colon cancer, and to reduce blood pressure.

Dairy products, including yogurt, cheese, and milk, are the most concentrated calcium sources going. A cup of milk and an equal amount of yogurt satisfies a three-year-old's daily calcium needs, while providing more than two-thirds of the calcium a four-, five-, or six-year-old requires. Plant foods such as broccoli, legumes (beans), and dark green leafy vegetables (but not spinach) provide calcium that is well absorbed by the body. Problem is, quantity counts. A three-year-old would need about 5 cups of cooked white beans or nearly the same amount of steamed broccoli to meet her daily calcium quota. What's more, milk is the only dairy food fortified with vitamin D, which promotes calcium uptake in the body and regulates bone and blood calcium levels.

Soy to the World

Soy protein holds promise for keeping blood cholesterol levels under control. That means clearer arteries, at least in adults. Soy also supplies isoflavones, plant substances that promote flexible arteries. Elastic arteries are better able to withstand daily wear and tear, especially with age. Soybeans are cholesterol-free, and so are most soy foods, including soy burgers, fresh and roasted soybeans, tofu, and tempeh. Soy products are suitable, protein-packed substitutes for meat, poultry, and seafood.

Food Rules

While scientific studies on the benefits of vitamin and mineral supplements are promising, researchers are often quick to point out that downing dietary supplements in the name of good health is not the same as eating a healthy diet. For instance, popping megadoses of beta-carotene, a powerful antioxidant nutrient that may ward off the cell damage that leads to heart disease and cancer, is not nearly as helpful as eating a carotenoid-rich diet. Why? Scientists suspect that the 500-plus members of the carotenoid family, which include lycopene, lutein, and zeaxanthin, probably work together to protect cells from damage. In fact, large-scale studies of the effects of supplemental beta-carotene have proved disappointing. The Institute of Medicine's Food and Nutrition Board says you cannot count on large doses of the antioxidant nutrients vitamins C and E, carotenoids, or the mineral selenium to ward off chronic disease.

Go for the Grain

Studies suggest eating whole grains lessens the risk for diabetes, high blood pressure, certain cancers, and heart disease. Scientists don't know exactly why whole grains are more beneficial than their highly refined counterparts, but it could be the combination of nutrients found in whole grains that's helpful, and not just the fiber they contain. Enriched whole grains such as oatmeal, brown rice, and whole-wheat pasta pack phytochemicals, fiber, minerals, and vitamins, most notably folic acid. Folic acid is a B vitamin that helps reduce the risk of certain birth defects, is needed for proper red blood cell development, and lowers blood levels of homocysteine. Excessive homocysteine in the bloodstream can increase the risk of heart disease and stroke, according to the American Heart Association.

A single serving of certain brands of fortified, enriched cereals can provide all the folic acid you or your child need for the day.

Brain Development: The Foundation for What Follows

Can the right mix of nutrients turn your daughter into a nuclear physicist, top-notch surgeon, or brilliant musician? It's not likely that nutrition confers smarts, but it does help maximize intellectual potential. Serving balanced meals and snacks should be part of a nurturing household that provides a supportive, smoke-free, nonviolent environment; this winning combination fosters peak brain development and encourages learning.

While good nutrition is no guarantee that your child will attend an Ivy League school or go on to obtain a Ph.D., there are ways of eating that maximize a child's genetic possibilities.

Setting Up the Circuitry

During gestation, the fetus develops hundreds of thousands of neurons every minute. Neurons are nerve cells responsible for communicating feelings, storing and retrieving memories, and processing information from the outside world, among other functions. Babies enter the world with billions of neurons, most of which stay with them for a lifetime. While the bulk of a baby's neurons are present at birth, the interconnections between them are sparse. That's one of the reasons why it takes months for a child to learn to talk, walk, and grab objects.

During the first two years of life, your baby's neurological development progresses at a frantic pace. During this time of critical brain development, neurons reach out to each other to form a vast communications network. While the circuitry in a baby's brain is becoming more complex, the body is busy "insulating" the wiring, as the brain goes through a critical stage of development called myelination. Myelin is the substance surrounding nerve cells. It provides the padding that prevents "short circuits" as information travels from one neuron to the next. Myelination actually begins during gestation and ends around eighteen months of age.

Nutrition Matters

Dozens of nutrients provide the foundation for peak brain function. In particular, a growing brain needs calories and protein for fuel and raw materials.

Here are some other nutrients considered vital to brain development.

Folic Acid. Taking folic acid, a B vitamin, is one of the ways a woman can help ensure proper brain development in her baby before she ever becomes pregnant. Folic acid helps prevent defects of the neural tube, a part of the body that evolves into the spinal cord and brain tissue. The neural tube begins developing within days after conception and is fully formed by about day thirty of the pregnancy. When the neural tube fails to close properly, spina bifida and anencephaly most often occur. Spina bifida is a defect of the lower part of the neural tube and may result in water on the brain and learning disabilities. Anencephaly is a fatal condition that results from incomplete formation of the upper portion of the neural tube. In anencephaly, the brain is absent or not fully formed.

Since many women don't realize they are expecting until after the most critical period of a baby's development, and because an estimated 50 percent of pregnancies are unplanned, health professionals recommend that all women capable of becoming pregnant take 400 micrograms of folic acid every day. Women who have had a baby with a neural tube defect need more folic acid and should consult their physician.

Fat. Fat helps babies flourish. You may strive to limit fat in your own diet, but babies need about 50 percent of their calories as fat for peak cognition. Breast milk is ideal for infants because it provides the right fat in the right amounts, changing with time to meet the needs of a developing infant.

Fat contains more than double the calories of carbohydrate and protein, making it useful as a concentrated energy source for a rapidly developing brain and body. Fat also supplies essential fatty acids (EFAs), the raw materials for cell building, particularly in the brain, which is about 60 percent fat by weight.

For brain growth, some fats may be better than others. Docosahexaenoic acid (DHA) and arachidonic acid (AA) are two polyunsaturated fatty acids that accumulate most rapidly in a developing baby's brain during the last trimester; they are equally important during infancy, too. Both are polyunsaturated fats that serve as raw materials for hormonelike compounds that foster peak nerve cell communication.

DHA is found primarily in fish but also in animals that eat fish products as part of their feed. The body makes AA from linoleic acid, which is found in nuts, seeds, and vegetable and seed oils such as corn oil or sunflower oil. Your child's body can also manufacture DHA from linolenic acid, which is concentrated in walnuts, wheat germ, flaxseed, canola oil, and soybean products.

Pregnant and nursing women who consume DHA-rich foods can increase their blood levels of this beneficial fat, making it available to their baby's developing brain tissue. In spite of its suspected importance in brain development, there is no official word on how much DHA expectant women, nursing mothers, and young children should consume. The U.S. Food and Drug Administration (FDA) does not require infant formula makers to add DHA, so formula-fed babies may not get DHA directly. Formulas in the United States contain linolenic acid, a fat that the body converts to DHA, albeit in limited amounts. The World Health Organization (WHO) recommends fortifying commercial infant formula with DHA.

While experts continue to debate the exact merits of DHA in humans, animal studies show that restricting DHA produces faulty visual function and diminished learning capacity. And a study published in *The Lancet* suggests that when DHA is added to infant formula, learning potential improves. The researchers found that babies who drank DHA-supplemented formula for the first four months of life performed better on problem-solving tests at ten months of age. Problem-solving tests are linked with IQ until at least age three.

Under the Sea

Fatty fish and animals that consume fish products are among the richest sources of DHA. Don't rely on DHA supplements for children who won't eat much of the following foods. There is no evidence that DHA supplements are safe or beneficial for your little one.

Top DHA sources:

- Beef
- Halibut
- Herring
- Lamb
- Mackerel*

- Salmon
- Sardines
- Trout
- Tuna

*The FDA advises that pregnant and nursing women and women capable of becoming pregnant avoid shark and swordfish, tilefish, and king mackerel. The recommendation stems from possible mercury poisoning. Mercury is a metal that easily crosses the placenta and can harm the nervous system of a developing fetus.

Freshwater fish may not be such a good idea for women in their childbearing years and for children, either. An eleven-year study at Wayne State University suggests a strong relationship between eating tainted fish from Lake Michigan and faulty brain development.

Choline. Choline is a vitamin that serves as the raw material for acetylcholine, a neurotransmitter that participates in a variety of brain and spinal cord functions and may improve memory and ability to learn. Neurotransmitters are the go-betweens for neurons, helping these nerve cells to communicate with each other. Nearly all of the scientific studies demonstrating the beneficial effects of choline involved animals, but researchers are hopeful that these positive findings apply to humans, too.

Don't look to your regular vitamin pill or prescription prenatal supplement for choline. They probably don't contain any, despite the fact that pregnancy and breastfeeding bump up choline requirements. That means pregnant women-and nursing moms-must consume choline from foods that are part of an otherwise well-balanced diet in order to make choline available to a developing baby. Eggs, meat, and peanuts are excellent choline sources. Choline is found in lesser amounts in a wide variety of foods, including iceberg lettuce, whole wheat bread, cauliflower, and tomato. Women who consume a diet with adequate calories and an array of foods should have little trouble meeting their choline needs.

Iron. Rapidly developing brain tissue requires a constant supply of oxygen. As part of red blood cells, iron is responsible for transporting oxygen to the brain. Iron is needed to make enzymes related to the production, function, and degradation of neurotransmitters, the brain's chemical messengers. In addition, the myelination process requires iron. During fetal development and well into the first two years of life, the body wraps nerve fibers in myelin to promote efficient communication. Low iron levels in the blood hamper the myelination of nerve cells, which can limit a child's cognitive abilities.

Because of its many vital functions, when infants and young children lack dietary iron, even for short periods, the effects on brain development may be irreversible. Iron deficiency during infancy can have long-term consequences for a child's ability to learn, possibly by reducing his attentiveness and responsiveness to the environment. Studies also show that children ages three to six who consume low-iron diets perform poorly on IQ tests, learning tests, and school achievement measures that indicate short-term memory, attention span, and tasks critical to solving visual problems.

LEAVE THESE BEHIND

What you avoid consuming is just as important as what you include when trying to maximize brain growth and cognitive powers.

Lead

Unborn babies and young children are particularly vulnerable to the effects of lead, which builds up in the body with time. Even a tiny amount can cause long-term developmental problems and learning disabilities in a child.

Depending on where you live, you could have lead in your drinking water. Dwellings constructed before 1986 may have plumbing that contains lead, which leaches into tap water. But even contemporary copper pipes may be joined by lead solder, with the same bad result for water lead levels.

Tap water isn't the only vehicle for lead, however. Fluids that sit in decanters and punch bowls made of lead crystal, and hot foods and beverages served in lead-glazed mugs and dishes, can increase lead levels in the body, too. Chipping lead paint and lead dust from renovations are highly concentrated sources of this very dangerous mineral.

Get the Lead Out

Protect your family against the effects of lead exposure with these tips.

- Call the Environmental Protection Agency (EPA) for information regarding certified labs in your state that can reliably test water lead levels. Reach the EPA at (800) 426-4791.
- Make sure your child gets enough iron in his diet. See page 30 for more on how much is enough. Children who consume adequate iron run a lower risk of lead poisoning should they be exposed to the mineral.
- Let the cold water run through your pipes for a minute or more before using tap water for drinking or for cooking. Running the faucet flushes out water that's been sitting in the pipes collecting lead.
- If you suspect lead in your pipes, opt for bottled water, which is typically lead free.
- Avoid chipping lead paint and any dwelling where lead paint removal or demolition is taking place.
- Think twice about burning candles in your home, as the wicks may contain lead that can be released in the air and be harmful to kids. Many U.S.–based candle makers do not use lead-core wicks, but it's difficult to determine lead content.

Alcohol

You probably know that it's a good idea to stay away from alcoholic beverages during pregnancy, but you may not realize just how smart it is.

Wine, beer, and spirits are the culprit in most cases of preventable mental retardation in the United States. Surprised? Don't be. Alcohol robs developing cells of oxygen, making normal development impossible. And the effects of alcohol on intellectual prowess are irreparable.

How much alcohol is too much? According to the March of Dimes, there is no known safe level of alcohol consumption in pregnancy. The March of Dimes also suggests avoiding alcohol when breastfeeding because it can slow the development of baby's motor skills, which allow her to walk and grab large objects. Likewise, the AAP cautions against alcohol since it can interfere with baby's ability to get milk from mom during nursing. Mother's drinking may also disturb an infant's sleep pattern, making her more wakeful and fussier.

Nutrition News: Take It with a Grain of Salt

Perhaps you find nutrition headlines intriguing and exciting. You want to hear about every new scientific finding, especially if it pertains to your child's health. Or maybe you are exposed to so much conflicting nutrition news that you tune it out to avoid confusion.

Either way, it pays to put nutrition findings into perspective. Even when a new study appears promising, it does not mean that you must immediately change your eating habits or the way your child eats.

Nutrition science is evolutionary, not revolutionary. Think of the scientific process as a road that is full of twists and turns—and pitfalls. A trip down this path is never linear. There are always dead ends to confront and some backtracking to be done. That's why no matter how definitive results look on paper (and in the headlines), the results of one or two studies do not automatically translate into eating recommendations. Rather, the results of a study, if conducted well and accepted as worthy by other qualified scientists, should become part of a larger pool of evidence, not usurp it.

Try to take the headlines about nutrition and health "discoveries" with cautious optimism. There's no harm in being interested, but before you alter your family's eating habits, find out more from a qualified health professional, such as a registered dietitian. Remember, it can take years or decades before experts agree on how much of a certain nutrient adults and children need.

The 10 Warning Signs of Junk Science

Wondering about a nutrition claim or the validity of the outcome of a "scientific" study? Put it to the test. If you can answer yes to any of these questions, chances are the claim or the study won't stand up to scientific scrutiny.

1. Does it promise a quick fix?
2. Are there dire warnings of danger regarding a single food product or dietary regimen?
3. Do the claims sound too good to be true?
4. Do they draw simplistic conclusions from a complex study?
5. Are eating recommendations based on a single study?
6. Are the statements refuted by reputable scientific organizations?
7. Are there lists of "good" and "bad" foods as part of the claim or the study?
8. Are there recommendations made to help sell a product?
9. Are there recommendations based on studies that are not reviewed by peers?
10. Are there recommendations from studies that ignore differences among individuals and groups?

Chapter 4

From Birth
to Four Months

Is she coming
home with us?

—Hayley, *age four*

BRINGING HOME BABY

They knew a sibling was on the way, but Hannah and Hayley could not have imagined that once she arrived, Emma would actually live with us, never mind how she would change their lives.

The first few months after a baby's arrival is a period of adjustment for every family member, especially older brothers and sisters. This is true no matter how many children you have.

As they strive to become accustomed to new routines that accommodate an infant, older children are also dealing with diminished attention from you and from other adult family members. Quite frankly, no one is getting the rest or the attention they crave, including Mom, who has the added task of recovering from the bodily changes produced by nine months of pregnancy and childbirth. Nursing moms must also be mindful of their diet and stress level in order to produce enough milk to nourish a newborn. Nursing or not, hormonal shifts and exhaustion tax limited emotional and physical resources.

Even in their exhausted state, experienced parents know that life will eventually settle down some, and that one day soon, they will actually sleep more and feel energetic again. So here's some advice for first-timers from a mom who has been there three times: Forget about the picture-perfect house and trying to hold it all together like you did before baby was born. Spend as much time as possible with your newborn, and devote time to taking care of yourself. The turmoil of the first few weeks and months may be overwhelming, but it passes and new family routines gradually take shape.

WHAT'S HAPPENING NOW: DEVELOPMENTAL MILESTONES

You've delivered your bundle of joy. Now what? Well, newborns generally sleep a lot. When he's not snoozing, your baby is usually eating, getting his diaper or outfit changed, or being cuddled by Mom, Dad, and other family members, or friends.

Babies crave physical contact. Touching your newborn a lot is especially crucial during the first six months of life. That's when babies form emotional bonds with parents and other loving adult caregivers such as grandparents and babysitters.

A child's future emotional development depends on the security of these early bonds.

Infants must learn to trust that their basic needs will be met again and again. Take eating as an example. Babies feel hunger pangs and begin to fuss and perhaps cry, a very distressing situation for them. Along comes an adult to relieve baby's discomfort, either by offering the breast or a bottle. The baby is relieved and in the bargain, he gets the chance to cuddle with another warm body, to listen to a soothing voice, and to study your face, as babies love to do. Breastfed babies get the added bonus of skin-to-skin contact.

As the hunger/feeding scenario is repeated anywhere from eight to twelve times a day, newborns begin to get the idea that Mom, Dad, or another person will provide what they need to make them feel content. This helps them to know that everything is OK in their world. Experts say that repeatedly satisfying an infant's physical and emotional needs creates feelings of security on a baby's part. Those feelings of trust provide the basis for the self-confidence that guides your child in trying out new things as he matures.

Four months marks a developmental milestone that influences how you feed your baby. It's the very first time that it's acceptable to serve infants solid food. Up until four months, the only nourishment newborns need is breast milk or commercial infant formula. Feeding baby solid foods before she's ready will not help her sleep better, contrary to what others might tell you. In fact, introducing solids early on can increase the risk of food allergies.

READ THIS BEFORE BABY ARRIVES

No matter how many parenthood prep classes you attend or how many books you read, there is nothing like real life to inform you about feeding a baby. Yet, one of the most crucial feeding decisions typically comes before your baby arrives. That's when parents ponder whether to feed baby infant formula or to breastfeed.

Don't worry if you don't know a lot about either way of nourishing your infant. Nobody is born with that knowledge, and up until now, you've had little reason to concern yourself with the subject. The time has come, however. Before baby arrives, investigate each feeding option. Carefully weigh the pros and cons of each so that you can decide what's right for you and your family.

You'll need some time to get familiar with breastfeeding or with infant formula. Couples choosing breastfeeding should attend a breastfeeding education class before delivery and brush up on the basics with a lactation consultant while in the hospital, if possible. Leave some time before you deliver to learn about breast pumps and to make an informed purchase. You'll also need to load up on nursing pads as part of your baby supplies.

Parents who decide on infant formula may want to check out the different kinds (see "Decisions, Decisions," page 85) and purchase some to have on hand when baby comes home. Don't forget to buy baby bottles and nipples. Educate yourself about preparing and handling infant formula.

In My Experience
Your Schedule or Mine?

While some babies quickly establish a feeding "routine" of sorts, infants typically go by an inner schedule that often mystifies their parents. Despite the annoying nighttime wake-up calls for comfort, it's wise to respond to your baby's cues to be fed or held at 2:00 A.M., rather than to try to make him conform to your need for order or for sleep. Forget the tired adage that picking up a newborn too often will spoil him. There's no reason in the world why a small baby should be allowed to wail. Why not? Babies cry to communicate. It's the only way they have to tell you that they need something. Newborns who are picked up promptly and cared for in a responsive way, including being fed on demand, often become contented beings as they head into their second six months of life, and beyond.

When baby needs to eat two times a night, it can be quite tiring for the new or experienced parent. Yet, when you try to get a newborn to feed according to your sleep schedule, it can backfire by interfering with her ability to fully develop the sense of trust she needs to flourish.

Does that mean around-the-clock parenting on your part is what it takes to have a happy, secure child? Not necessarily. There's no reason why any parent should do all the work when there is another adult to shoulder some of the load. For example, delegating feeding duties cuts Mom's stress. Dad can give baby a bottle during the night just as easily as Mom can provide the breast. For all three of our children, my husband encouraged me to pump enough milk so that he could feed the baby during the night a couple of times a week. For me, those few hours of uninterrupted sleep boosted my sagging energy levels and gave me the stamina to be a better parent during the day.

Friends, relatives, and, yes, complete strangers will try to sway you to one feeding option or the other. Forget what others say about the way babies should eat. You should choose the method that's right for you, but only after considering all of the pros and cons regarding breastfeeding and infant formula. Likewise, refrain from transferring your experience with feeding your other children to this baby. For example, if you had difficulty nursing your first child, don't assume that you'll experience difficulties this time around as well.

There's no reason to believe that you cannot breastfeed a baby just because your others got formula. I'll never forget the couple in the breastfeeding education class I attended before Hayley was born. They came to learn the basics of breast-feeding so that the mom could nurse their third child. Even though the couple chose formula for their first two children, they were committed to breastfeeding the third. I don't know how it turned out for them, but I suspect it went well because they were open to breastfeeding without being fearful of it.

Can you change your mind about what to feed your baby after she's born? Perhaps. Plenty of women begin with breastfeeding and switch to infant formula. But it doesn't usually work the other way around. So if you're entertaining any thoughts of breastfeeding, I urge you to give it a try. A detailed explanation of breastfeeding and its myriad benefits begins on page 69.

BETTING ON BREASTFEEDING

> *Hannah, then age three: "Mummy, what are you doing?"*
> *Me: "I'm feeding the baby."*
> *Hannah: "Yuck!"*

That conversation took place the day after I delivered our third child, Emma. The girls were visiting the hospital along with my husband and mother. The baby was hungry, so I began to nurse her. As I did, the older girls gaped in surprise. That's when Hannah weighed in on breastfeeding. We adults had a good laugh about Hannah's remark, and the memory of her reaction still makes me smile nearly two years later.

As Hannah and Hayley became accustomed to my nursing Emma, I would often point out that a mother's body is perfectly designed to feed a baby. In trying to figure out breastfeeding, the girls would pose all sorts of different questions, including: Does it hurt? How do you make milk? and Where does the milk come out?

No doubt, you have your own questions about breastfeeding, particularly if you're contemplating nursing a baby for the first time. Don't feel embarrassed by your lack of nursing knowledge. Knowing how to breastfeed is not the same thing as knowing how to make your mother's pot roast recipe. Generally speaking, our mothers and grandmothers did not breastfeed, because it was largely discouraged at the time. Unfortunately, that limits our information sources about the benefits of nursing, never mind the practical aspects of how to actually breastfeed a baby.

> ## In My Experience
> ### Call in a Consultant
>
> Moms new to nursing a baby (and even experienced breastfeeding women) need all the encouragement they can get. If you're having any sort of difficulty with breastfeeding, you need a caring, knowledgeable expert to provide advice and to cheer you on. Certified lactation consultants are just the ticket. After having some trouble with pain and improper positioning during the initial weeks of nursing my first child, I paid for a home visit by a lactation consultant whom I had met in the hospital. Getting together with Michelle for an hour was one of the smartest moves I have made to date as a parent. She assured me that I was doing a good job, and that my problems would soon be resolved. That cheered me up and gave me the necessary confidence to go on breastfeeding Hayley and two more children after her.
>
> Hospital-based breastfeeding classes are a boon, but you may run into problems when you get home. When you need help, rely on International Board Certified Lactation Consultants (IBCLCs). As health care professionals who meet the eligibility requirements set by the International Board of Lactation Consultant Examiners, members possess the knowledge and positive attitude needed to provide quality breastfeeding advice for nursing moms and their babies. IBCLCs work in hospitals, community settings, and in private practice.

Breastfeeding Benefits

Without question, breastfeeding is best for baby. Breast milk is one of nature's most perfectly designed foods. It contains all the right nutrients in the correct amounts to foster baby's brain development and physical growth for about the first six months of his life. Breast milk is tailored to meet your baby's needs, and its nutrient composition evolves to accommodate his growth.

Several health organizations, including the American Dietetic Association and the AAP, recommend nursing a baby for at least a year (longer if desired). The AAP encourages Mom to breastfeed exclusively until baby reaches six months of age. You may think these are lofty breastfeeding goals that most mothers are unlikely to achieve. But please don't be put off. Any amount of breastfeeding is better than none. Even a few months of nursing while on maternity leave counts toward your baby's good health. That may come as a happy surprise to women who are planning to switch over to infant formula once they return to work. Working does not have to interfere with breastfeeding, however. Many women nurse their children in the morning and at night and pump their milk to be fed to baby from a bottle when they are not around. That way, baby reaps the benefits of breast milk while being cared for by a sitter.

Breastfeeding:

- Inspires maternal confidence. It's wonderful to see how baby thrives from the milk Mom's body produces. It's one of the greatest miracles of life.
- Is a one-of-a-kind opportunity for Mom and baby to bond. Your infant can snuggle up close to you while receiving the nurturing he needs in the way of food and physical contact.
- Is a money-saver. You may need to eat some additional food to keep up your milk production, but food costs don't come close to the price of infant formula, which the AAP puts at upwards of $1,000 for the first year.
- Is convenient and saves time. Your baby's food supply is always with Mom. There's no shopping for and preparing formula and no water, bottles, and nipples to clean every day, either.
- Promotes better digestion and quicker maturation of the intestinal tract. Breast milk is easier for baby to digest than infant formula. It provides substances that ensure that an infant's body properly breaks down the protein and fat in breast milk.
- Helps Mom's uterus get back in shape faster, protects against breast cancer, and keeps blood pressure in check. As baby sucks on the breast, the hormone oxytocin makes its way into Mom's bloodstream. Oxytocin prompts the uterus to shrink to its regular size, and more. Researchers at the University of North Carolina at Chapel Hill found that nursing promotes blood pressure control, and they credit oxytocin for inducing calm. According to the American Medical Association (AMA), nursing a baby for at least three months reduces your chance of developing breast cancer later in life.
- Lowers the rates of allergy and asthma, diabetes, digestive tract infection, and respiratory and ear infections in babies. That's not to say that nursing guarantees immunity. Many other factors contribute to your child's susceptibility and contact with germs, including siblings, day care, and pacifiers, which can convey germs by coming in contact with unclean surfaces and hands.
- May reduce your baby's chances for cardiovascular disease in adulthood. At least one study, published in the *Archives of Diseases in Childhood*, found that babies who were exclusively breastfed for at least ten days had fewer of the risk factors for cardiovascular disease some fifty-plus years after birth.

- May foster weight control later in life. German researchers have found that five- and six-year-olds who were nursed the longest as babies before beginning formula or food were far less likely to be overweight.
- Enhances baby's brain function and fosters peak eyesight. Breast milk supplies two fats, AA and DHA, found lacking in cow's milk. AA and DHA are associated with improved cognitive powers and well-developed vision. The longer you breastfeed, the greater the effects on your child's mental acumen, motor abilities, and vision. Mom's diet can influence the amount of AA and DHA available to baby's brain by way of breast milk. See page 57 for more.
- Promotes softer, sweeter-smelling stools than those of formula-fed infants.
- Reduces health care costs. A study done by the University of Arizona Department of Pediatrics found that exclusively breastfed babies had a lower incidence of ear infections, respiratory infections such as colds, and intestinal infections. That meant fewer doctor's visits, hospitalizations, and costly prescriptions than for formula-fed children.
- Helps lower leukemia risk in children. A *Journal of the National Cancer Institute* report found that breastfed infants might have a lower risk of developing some forms of childhood leukemia than their bottle-fed counterparts. The longer children nursed, the greater the protection.

Overcoming Breastfeeding Barriers

You're considering breastfeeding, but you're just not sure it's right for you. Perhaps you've heard nursing horror stories that make you want to run to the nearest store to stock up on formula. Maybe you fed formula to your other children, and now you're considering breastfeeding this baby.

In the end, you must do what's best for you and your family. But first, you need the facts to make an informed decision. Here's some straight talk about breastfeeding that I hope will help.

Barrier: You think that you may flunk breastfeeding.

Solution: You're afraid, and that's to be expected. But you can't fail at something you've never tried. Stop listening to friends and relatives that did not have a good experience with nursing. Stick with health professionals and seasoned breastfeeding pros, including experienced mothers, who can provide you with facts while offering support.

Barrier: You have to work at breastfeeding.

Solution: It may be a natural function, but it doesn't always come naturally at the start (neither did toilet training). Both you and baby will probably go through a period of adjustment as you learn the breastfeeding basics, but it's worth it. Many babies and their moms get the hang of nursing soon after birth and go on to have a successful relationship that lasts for months afterward.

Barrier: You are concerned about producing enough milk.

Solution: Not to worry. The more you nurse, the more milk you make. Some women do not have enough glandular tissue to produce adequate milk to nourish their babies, but this condition is rare. Even if you think you are small breasted and can't produce enough milk, don't be concerned. Your breasts can make just as much milk as larger ones.

Barrier: Inverted or flat nipples.

Solution: Many times, inverted or flat nipples don't hinder breastfeeding. Wearing breast shields during your third trimester and between feedings once the baby is born may help, so ask your doctor about this.

Barrier: Breastfeeding is messy.

Solution: Nursing is not always a tidy business. Let's be frank. Your breasts leak, and they are capable of shooting milk clear across the room! When does that happen? When a baby suckling at the breast suddenly stops but your milk flow continues. Invest in lots of breast pads to take care of any leaks, and wear appropriate clothing, that is, two layers, to disguise minor leaks. Each time you nurse, have on hand a cloth or towel you won't mind getting wet. Cloth diapers work well to clean up during and after nursing.

Barrier: Breastfeeding hurts.

Solution: Nursing may be a bit uncomfortable at the start because your breasts are not accustomed to a baby's powerful suckling. I had this problem a couple of times, and I used acetaminophen, patience, and perseverance to overcome it. The initial pain you may have with breastfeeding should go away within days to a week, however. In the meantime, ask your licensed health care provider about over-the-counter pain relievers to alleviate the discomfort. If breast pain persists, improper positioning is most likely the cause, although there may be other reasons. Here's why: Your baby gets milk by pressing on the areola, the dark area surrounding the nipple, not from the nipple itself. Baby must be encouraged to open her mouth very wide to get as much of the areola into her mouth as possible. If she doesn't open wide enough, she will end up suckling on the nipple, and you will end up in pain.

Mastitis could also be a source of breast pain. It's a bacterial infection that usually develops in just one of your breasts. You feel tired and achy, like you've got the flu. You do not have to stop nursing, however. In fact, breastfeeding helps clear up the infection by draining the breast. You doctor may prescribe antibiotics that are safe to take during nursing.

The absence of fever combined with reduced milk flow and a sore breast may mean you have a plugged milk duct rather than mastitis. Breast tenderness may be treatable by massaging the affected area, frequent nursing, and applying moist heat. In any case, call your doctor immediately.

Barrier: Breastfeeding is a lot of responsibility for Mom.

Solution: You may be the sole food provider, but you are not the only one capable of feeding the baby. Purchase a breast pump before baby is born, and read up on how to use it. Wait a couple of weeks or more after delivery to begin pumping milk. Allow your infant to get accustomed to taking small amounts of expressed breast milk by having your husband, partner, or other adult give your newborn milk from a baby bottle. Forget about the dire warnings that baby will become confused about how to suck on the bottle's nipple and your own. Taking the chance that he won't become confused buys you some much-needed freedom. Expressing milk and allowing others to feed my girls helped me think more positively about nursing, which perpetuated breastfeeding in my case.

Barrier: Breastfeeding in public can be difficult, uncomfortable, and embarrassing.

Solution: Some people are offended when they see women feeding their baby the way nature intended. Truth is, you may want to be more discreet, but it's not always possible. Very few public places provide private spaces for nursing moms. Whenever I brought the kids to a nearby mall, I would silently curse the mall management for overlooking the fact that nursing mothers would like to be more comfortable when breastfeeding (although it did not stop me from going out with all three kids in tow). You can avoid embarrassment by covering up with a towel or receiving blanket when nursing in public, feeding the baby in the parking lot before going into a mall or restaurant, or requesting a more private booth or table when dining out.

WHEN NURSING IS NOT AN OPTION

Despite its benefits, breastfeeding is not always the smartest feeding choice. If you or your baby have a chronic medical condition, formula feeding could be best. Women who use illicit drugs or who take certain prescription and over-the-counter medications on a daily basis should check with their obstetrician and pediatrician about the safety of nursing their babies. Here are some of the situations that preclude breastfeeding.

HIV and other infectious diseases: Human immunodeficiency virus (HIV) is the virus that causes acquired immunodeficiency syndrome (AIDS). HIV can be transmitted from mother to child through breast milk. Experts at the Centers for Disease Control and Prevention recommend women who test positive for the HIV antibody not breastfeed their baby. Moms with T-cell leukemia virus infection or untreated tuberculosis should also avoid breastfeeding to reduce risk of transmission to baby.

Chemotherapy and other medications: Women receiving chemotherapy and certain other medications for chronic illness should not breastfeed. A number of drugs that are unsafe for a developing baby are passed on through breast milk.

Illicit drug use: Moms who use any amount of marijuana, cocaine, heroine, or any other recreational drug should avoid nursing.

WHAT TO EXPECT: THE FIRST TWO WEEKS

I've always thought that the first two weeks of nursing were the hardest to deal with, whether it was my first baby or my third. Once I was over that two-week hump, it seemed that nursing was, with a few exceptions, smooth sailing.

It takes about two weeks to establish a routine with baby, which changes often because of growth spurts, the first of which occurs between eight and twelve days. Subsequent surges in development that prompt baby to feed more frequently take place at about three to four weeks, and again at three months or so. After that, growth spurts are variable.

The more you know, the better you will be able to handle breastfeeding during this critical time when you are more likely to throw in the towel because you don't think you're doing it right. Here's what to expect from moments after delivery.

In the Delivery Room

Within the first two hours or so after birth, babies seek comfort in their mother's breast. Their instinct is to latch on and suck, so right after delivery is typically the best time to first nurse your baby. If you can't feed the baby soon after birth, make it clear to the delivery room staff and to the nursery personnel that you want to breastfeed as soon as possible, and that you don't want the baby to receive any supplemental feedings of formula or water if it's not medically necessary. Supplemental infant formula can confuse a baby just learning to nurse, because sucking on artificial nipples uses different tongue and jaw motions than does suckling at the breast. Have the baby stay with you if possible. This arrangement, called rooming in, encourages breastfeeding and reduces the odds that your baby will get supplemental feedings.

Sometimes women have a difficult delivery or their baby is born with certain problems that prevent breastfeeding right after birth. Does that mean breastfeeding becomes impossible? Not necessarily. My friend Hillary's situation beautifully illustrates that point.

Hillary delivered a son who was immediately whisked away to the Neonatal

Intensive Care Unit. Because he required help breathing, her baby was placed on a respirator, ruling out breastfeeding for the time being. That didn't deter Hillary, however. While she waited for her baby to get well enough to breath on his own, she pumped her milk. Three days after delivery, Hillary first nursed her son, and it went without a hitch. Nine months later, he's a happy, robust boy who has clearly benefited from breastfeeding and the commitment his mother made to nursing.

Jaundice and Breastfeeding

Here's another reason to make sure hospital staff don't feed your baby sterile water or sugar-water supplements when you're not looking. According to the AAP, supplemental feedings of water can boost bilirubin levels in baby's bloodstream. High bilirubin counts may cause jaundice, which, left untreated, can result in brain damage. In fact, breast milk (and infant formula) can help prevent jaundice. Why? Bilirubin is eliminated in baby's bowel movements, and it takes breast milk or infant formula to form the stool.

The First Couple of Days

Baby may want to nurse, but the truth is, there's little for him to eat, largely because your milk hasn't "come in" yet. Don't despair, your newborn's belly is tiny and his nutrient needs are minimal for the first few days. And what you have to offer him—colostrum—is packed with exactly what he needs.

Colostrum is the highly nutritious liquid your breasts make right before they begin producing milk in earnest, which is about two to five days after delivery. Colostrum is rich in protective white blood cells and antibodies that ward off infection. Colostrum also coats baby's digestive tract to help prevent absorption of harmful substances by the body. As far as nutrition goes, colostrum contains concentrated amounts of protein, is relatively low in carbohydrate and fat, and is easy to digest.

Infants snooze a lot just after birth, but they should not be allowed to sleep through feedings. Newborns may be sluggish, but they must nurse at least eight to twelve times in a twenty-four-hour period and should take milk for about ten to twenty minutes from each breast. It's important to try to empty each breast so that baby can reap the benefits of hind milk, the fattiest, most calorie-dense milk, which comes later in the feeding. Wake sleepy babies every three hours or so by unwrapping their blanket, loosening their clothes, or gently wiping their face with a warm, wet cloth. Switching breasts can boost a tired baby's interest in feeding. It also promotes even milk production in each breast, which helps cut down on engorgement, best described as milk buildup.

Days Three Through Five

As your milk production picks up, chances are your breasts will feel rock hard, tender, and warm to the touch. Frequent nursing—as mentioned above—actually relieves the pressure and general discomfort from milk buildup. Eventually, this normal engorgement will pass, usually after the first few days or so of nursing. There is an irony in engorgement: the harder your breasts, the tougher it is for the baby to latch on properly. Pumping or expressing milk by hand makes breasts soft enough so that baby can latch on. Sometimes gently massaging the breast while baby is feeding provides relief, too. If engorgement doesn't resolve itself within two days, call your health care provider.

When it's time to feed baby again, start with the breast you ended with at the previous feeding. One good way of remembering which breast to begin with is by attaching a safety pin to the strap of your nursing bra on the side where you should start feeding the baby.

If your baby doesn't latch on correctly to the breast, it can be painful, never mind counterproductive. Chronic breast pain causes stress and may make you want to quit breastfeeding because you don't think you're doing it right.

To release milk from the breast, babies must suck on the areola, not the nipple. As baby latches on to the breast, she activates what's known as the let-down reflex. Suckling signals the body to release oxytocin, a hormone that prompts contractions of the breast tissue, allowing the milk to make it down to the nipple for baby to drink. Let-down is a great relief for moms and is characterized by tingling or warmth in breast as the milk begins to flow.

How will you know nursing is going well? Listen and watch for baby's swallowing while feeding. Don't fret if your baby sucks a few times and then rests, because it's perfectly normal. Clucking noises or dimples in her cheeks probably mean she isn't getting enough milk from the breast. Try repositioning. Use your pinkie to break the hold she has on your breast. When she goes to latch on again, make sure she opens wide, that her lower lip does not curl under, and that she's taking in the areola. Another positive sign of successful breastfeeding is in your baby's diapers. By her third day of life, your newborn will probably have had three to four wet diapers and one to two stools that are beginning to take on a yellow appearance. As long as your daughter is content after finishing a feeding and is gaining weight according to your pediatrician, then she is probably nursing just fine.

Many mothers worry that their babies are not getting enough nourishment from breast milk alone. Granted, there are times when this may be true, but in most cases, a lack of confidence in your milk supply is unjustified. Here's why. The more you feed your baby, the more milk you make. Giving baby supplemental formula without expressing your own milk serves to stymie milk production. There are cases when breastfed babies require water or infant formula, but they are few and far between. Before you feed your child anything but breast milk, or if you are experiencing any problems with your newborn, call your pediatrician.

A LATCH MADE IN HEAVEN

Positioning is everything in breastfeeding. If your baby doesn't latch on correctly, nursing will not last for long.

Breastfeeding is a natural function, and most babies know what to do intuitively. Chances are, your child will be eager to begin suckling soon after birth. But don't be surprised if you both need a little help getting started, especially if you've had a long and difficult delivery or baby is not hungry right after being born. Learning to latch on may take a bit of time and patience, but you'll both soon get the hang of it.

There are three positions you may use to feed your baby: cradle hold, football hold, and lying down. Try the cradle hold to learn how to latch on properly. Get comfortable in bed with pillows to support your back, or in a chair. Place baby in the crook of your arm, rotating his entire body toward you. Bring baby's head up to your breast. Check to see that he is facing straight toward you and that his head, chest, and abdomen are all aligned. Using the opposite hand, take one of your breasts and tickle baby's lips lightly with your nipple. Stroking his lips with the nipple stimulates the rooting reflex, and he is inclined to open wide to get the breast in his mouth. Use your other arm to cradle baby and support his head.

Now comes the tricky part. Once baby's mouth is fully open, swiftly bring him to the breast. Your baby's instinct will tell him to latch on and begin nursing. Avoid the urge to lean closer to baby to get the breast in his mouth. It's tempting to go to baby, rather than bring baby to you, but it causes you to hunch over, which could lead to back strain.

How do you know baby's on the breast the right way? Pain can be your guide. The goal is getting baby to compress the areola (the dark area around the nipple) to get milk, not to nurse from your nipple. In fact, your nipple needs to be in the back of baby's mouth during nursing in order for him to correctly compress the areola and activate milk flow. The correct latch will be fairly tight, and you can check correct positioning by looking to see whether most of the areola is in baby's mouth. If nursing hurts, chances are your baby is latching on to the nipple. This is a sign to remove the baby and reposition. Gently insert your pinkie finger into your baby's mouth to break his grip on the breast and begin again.

FINDING THE PERFECT POSITION

Once you've mastered latching on, it really doesn't matter which of the three most common nursing positions you use. I was a fan of the cradle and football holds for my first two girls. But once Emma came along, I was too tired to sit up, especially at night. That's when I began lying down to breastfeed most of the time.

Each position has advantages. For example, I got a lot of reading done when nursing sitting up, but a lot more rest when I did it lying down. Don't forget to nurse from both breasts no matter which position you choose.

Cradle

The cradle position is rather self-explanatory: Your baby lies in the crook of your arm, which you use to move her around to get close to your breast. Sit up with plenty of support for your back. I also put a pillow on my lap to help lessen the strain on the arm that I was using to cradle the baby. A lap pillow also helps when you are switching sides, as it provides a soft place for baby to take a short time-out between breasts.

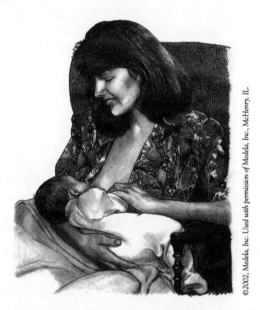

©2002, Medela, Inc. Used with permission of Medela, Inc., McHenry, IL.

Football

I think this position offers more control when trying to get baby to latch on properly, largely because you can better guide his head. To begin, you'll need at least two pillows. Place one pillow on your lap and the other pillow to the side of you. Put the baby on your lap with his legs pointing toward your back, keeping your hand under his head and back for support. Make sure his mouth is level with your nipple before you begin. This is a great position for nursing twins because you can feed two simultaneously. It's also good after cesarean delivery since it keeps pressure off your abdomen.

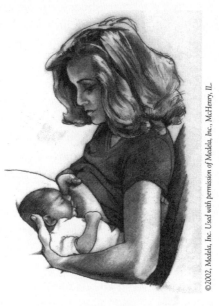

©2002, Medela, Inc. Used with permission of Medela, Inc., McHenry, IL.

Lying Down

This position was invented for tired moms! Begin by lying next to baby on the side you want to nurse on. Turn baby to face you, making sure his mouth is level with your nipple while you support his head and back with your free arm. This is a great nursing position for women recovering from a cesarean birth.

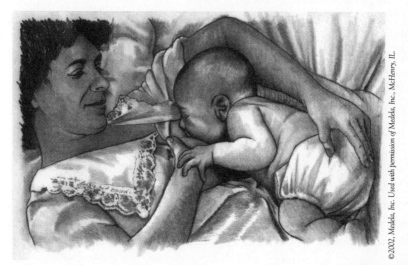

©2002, Medela, Inc. Used with permission of Medela, Inc., McHenry, IL.

TIME OUT FOR MOM

With all that you have to do in a day, it's easy to see why you put taking care of yourself at the bottom of the list. Yet, ignoring your needs is actually counterproductive, especially for nursing mothers. Successful breastfeeding depends largely on how Mom treats herself. A poor diet, too little sleep, and too much stress can reduce the quality and quantity of your milk supply. Here are the basics of self-care for postpartum women.

Ask for help. When in doubt, reach out. Call on friends and family to help reduce your anxiety in any way possible. Lactation consultants and the staff at your pediatrician's office should be able to solve your breastfeeding problems and answer your questions, no matter how silly you think your concerns are.

Take care of your breasts. Nursing moms should avoid using soap on nipples or the areola when taking a shower or bath and should stay away from lanolin or antiseptics. Purchase sturdy cotton nursing bras with flaps that easily expose the breast and can unhook and reattach easily with one hand. Whenever possible, especially in the beginning, let breasts air-dry for five to ten minutes to prevent chafing and subsequent irritation. Always change your bra if it becomes wet with milk.

Get some R & R. Forget about all nonessential housework. Don't try to fold laundry or clean the bathroom while baby is napping. You must rest, too. Cut down on answering phone calls by communicating via e-mail and using your answering machine. That's what technology is for! Snooze or rest when baby does, especially if you are getting very little uninterrupted sleep at night. Whenever I could, I turned off the phone ringer, pulled down the shades, nursed the baby, and then napped in the middle of the day.

Eat right. Nursing or not, you need to keep up your energy, which includes eating the right amount of healthy foods and continuing to take a multivitamin with iron to replenish what's lost during delivery as part of blood. New moms should not restrict their calories until at least six weeks after delivery. Women who do not nurse their babies should eat at least 1,600 calories a day to help their bodies return to normal; breastfeeding moms eating fewer than 1,800 calories daily can jeopardize milk production (see "Your Breastfeeding Diet," page 81).

Move it, but take care. Physical activity relieves stress and can help you fit into your prepregnancy clothes faster. But before you lace up your running shoes, you need a doctor's OK, which typically comes at your six-week postpartum checkup. Even then, take it slow. Make exercise a family affair by taking baby with you on walks. Or work out at home with specially designed videotapes for postpartum fitness.

Stop before you pop. Nursing moms need to avoid all drugs, including over-the-counter medications that have not been approved by a licensed health care professional.

YOUR BREASTFEEDING DIET

When you're her sole source of nutrition, what you eat affects your baby's health and development. Sometimes, nurturing a baby is done at your expense, however. According to a study in the *Journal of the American Dietetic Association*, breast-feeding women lacked adequate calcium; vitamins B_6, D, and E; folic acid; and zinc because they did not eat right when nursing. That doesn't need to be the case, however. You're feeding two people, so you should focus on consuming a balanced diet while keeping the following in mind.

Calories. Nursing a baby requires more energy than a pregnancy. To make enough milk, you must eat about 500 additional calories every day (in pregnancy, it was 300). Most women will need about 2,700 calories daily to produce adequate amounts of milk for their babies. If you're thinking of fitting into your prepregnancy clothes, no doubt weight loss is on your mind. Go slow. You'll need at least 1,800 calories a day to continue breastfeeding. Eating fewer calories can decrease milk production. If you're dropping more than four pounds a month, increase your calories to adequately nourish yourself and your baby simultaneously.

Fat. Nursing babies require docosahexanoic acid (DHA) and arachidonic acid (AA), two fats that foster brain development and peak vision. To get enough of these vital fats, include fatty fish such as salmon twice weekly, and make nuts, green leafy vegetables, soy products, and vegetable seed oils such as sunflower and canola oils a part of your daily diet. Fattier fish are the most concentrated food sources of DHA, but any fish will do, especially if you don't like the stronger tasting varieties. Avoid shark, swordfish, king mackerel, and tilefish because of potentially dangerous mercury levels.

Fluid. Breast milk is 87 percent water, so milk production means drinking more fluid. You probably won't have any trouble downing enough milk, juice, or water, since you will be thirsty. Don't wait until thirst hits to drink, however. As a breastfeeding mother, you need a total of close to 100 ounces or twelve 8-ounce glasses of fluid daily. Here's a tip: Pour yourself a glass of water each time you sit down to nurse to help keep up with fluid loss. Avoid caffeinated beverages, since caffeine makes its way into breast milk and can interfere with baby's sleep. Stay away from alcohol, too. There's evidence that alcohol in breast milk affects a baby's motor skills and sleep patterns.

Choline. Choline is key to your infant's brain development, so make sure to include choline-rich foods such as eggs and beef in your diet on a regular basis. Meat is an excellent source of iron, too.

Supplements. Finish off your prenatal vitamin/mineral supplement, then switch to a multivitamin with iron that provides at least 400 micrograms of folic acid and 100 percent of the Daily Value (DV) for iron. Avoid herbal supplements and other botanicals. There's no proof that they are safe for nursing babies.

BACK TO WORK

Good news: Successful breastfeeding and working do mix. As long as there is a private place for you to pump at work and reliable refrigeration for expressed milk, it's relatively simple to continue providing baby with the benefits of breast milk for as long as possible, even while you're on the job.

Express yourself. Practice pumping at home (see "Choosing a Breast Pump," below), beginning two weeks before you return to work. That leaves you plenty of time to become acquainted with expressing milk and allows baby to get accustomed to drinking your milk from a bottle instead of directly from you. Pump at work every three hours or so, more often if you feel the need. Promptly refrigerate or freeze expressed milk.

Baby, meet Mr. Bottle. Wait at least two weeks after delivery before offering a bottle to your newborn, but don't delay the introduction until just days before returning to work. Waiting until the last minute could mean that baby refuses the bottle, and then you're in trouble. Have another person, such as your husband or partner, a babysitter, or a grandparent, offer bottles to your baby, beginning two weeks before you return to your job.

Timing is everything. On work days, breastfeed your baby just before you leave the house and when you get home. Chances are, this will take some doing. You may have to wake up earlier to make sure that you can get ready to go out and still have the time to feed the baby. Depending on your schedule and when your day care provider gives baby a bottle, you can nurse right when you get home, before your baby's bedtime, or both.

Plan ahead. On the evening before a workday, pack everything you need to pump milk on the job. Don't forget to take along a healthy lunch and snack. That way, you won't waste time rounding up food or equipment in the morning.

Choosing a Breast Pump

Consider your needs. Most pumps are portable, efficient, and easy to use. How often you intend to pump dictates the durability of the pump you need. In turn, durability drives cost. Bottom line: the more durable, the more you can pump, but the costlier the machine.

Collecting, Storing, and Handling Breast Milk

At home or at work, there are certain guidelines to follow when using a breast pump and handling expressed breast milk.

- Wash your hands well with warm soapy water before starting.
- Make sure all of your breast pump equipment is clean from the last time you pumped.
- The best time to pump is midway between feedings. If your son or daughter skips a feeding or skimps on one, express the remaining milk in the breast for later use. When you're away from the baby all day, pump every three hours or so to keep up milk production.
- You can store pumped milk in a number of ways. When I pumped at work, I would express milk directly into a small baby bottle, and then seal it and refrigerate it. I toted the milk home in a cooler bag. Once home, I placed the milk in the refrigerator to bring to my babysitter the next day. When I pumped at home to stockpile milk for when I was away from my children, I preferred plastic bags for freezing milk I wouldn't use within a day or so. You pump into the bottle that comes with your pump, then transfer the milk to storage bags such as Gerber's Seal 'n Go Breast Milk Storage Bags. Don't forget to record the date and amount before refrigerating or freezing breast milk.

   Refrigerated fresh breast milk is good for up to forty-eight hours as long as your refrigerator registers 39°F or slightly below. (Get a thermometer if you're in doubt.) To freeze breast milk, leave some space at the top of the container, as breast milk expands as it freezes. Always mark the date and use the oldest milk first. Frozen milk is good for up to two weeks. Place breast milk in the back of the freezer for maximum coldness; don't place it on the door since it may not freeze to the proper temperature. Freeze in small portions so that you won't waste breast milk, and never refreeze thawed breast milk. Discard any milk that you don't use during a feeding. Freezing does not significantly alter either the nutrients or the immunological components in breast milk.

(continued)

- For quick thaw, place frozen breast milk in a bowl of warm water and wait a few minutes, then gently swirl to promote melting and to mix any fat that may have separated and stuck to the sides of the container. Always test a drop of milk on the inside of your wrist to make sure the milk won't burn baby's mouth. Use refrigerated, thawed breast milk within twenty-four hours.
- Never microwave breast milk. It decreases the nutrients and raises the possibility of burning your baby's mouth.

Manual, or hand-operated, pumps can cost the least amount of money and are the most useful for women who pump on an occasional basis. Electric pumps depend on batteries or AC adapters for their power supply. Automatic electric pumps tend to appeal to women who must express larger volumes of milk in a limited time frame, such as working women and mothers of premature babies. While costlier, some of these efficient pumps can express milk from both breasts simultaneously, which cuts your pumping time by half.

Does Baby Need Extra Vitamins and Minerals?

Every infant requires a vitamin K supplement at birth to prevent a bleeding disorder. Experts say healthy breastfed infants typically do not need any other supplemental vitamins or minerals with a few exceptions. Dark-skinned infants require extra vitamin D when they are exclusively breastfed, especially if they don't get much strong summer sunlight. Ditto for heavily clad babies whose skin doesn't see much sun. Why? Summer sunlight sparks vitamin D production in the body.

There is no need to give nursing infants supplemental iron until four to six months of age. That's when their own iron stores become depleted. Breastfed babies do not require fluoride supplements during their first six months but may need them thereafter if the water they drink is deficient in fluoride.

FORMULA FEEDING

Many babies in the United States receive nourishment by way of infant formula, either in place of breast milk or in addition to it. Formula provides a certain element of freedom for parents and other caregivers, particularly because any adult is capable of feeding the baby at any time, precluding mom as the sole food source.

Formula is beneficial for other reasons, too.

- Some infants cannot tolerate the carbohydrate or protein in breast milk and depend upon specialized infant formula for survival.
- Moms who cannot breastfeed for one reason or the other (see page 73) rely on infant formula as a suitable substitute.
- Premature or low-birth-weight infants (under 5.5 pounds) and full-term babies who don't gain enough weight on breast milk alone often improve when infant formula is added to their diet.

Decision, Decisions

Infant formula makers try to come as close as possible to copying the composition of mother's milk. However, it's impossible to completely duplicate human milk, given its hundreds of different components. Even so, babies do thrive on infant formula. I did, and chances are, you did, too.

Still, there are some major nutritional differences between breast milk and formula. Generally speaking, formula contains more protein. Vitamin and mineral content can be higher, too, often to compensate for the possible lower rate of absorption of these nutrients from the formula.

Certain infant formulas are touted as low iron, yet there is rarely a medical need for low-iron formulas. In fact, inadequate iron intake can harm brain development and overall growth. That's why the AAP is against using low-iron infant formulas. Never feed your baby a low-iron formula without the approval of your pediatrician.

Form, Not Function, Is the Difference

Infant formula comes in three forms: ready-to-feed, concentrated liquid, and powder. Price and convenience, not nutrition, are what differentiates them from each other.

Convenience is costly. That's why powdered formulas are the cheapest of all. Aside from the price break, powdered formula has other advantages, particularly for breastfeeding moms who want to supplement their milk supply. You can mix as much of the powdered formula as you need, without waste. Powdered formula preparation is more time consuming than that of the other, costlier, forms. You must measure the formula carefully, as well as boil the water to mix with it. Powders have a thirty-day shelf life after opening.

The two types of liquid formula vary in concentration and cost. Concentrated liquid formula is meant to be mixed with an equal part of boiled water and delivered to baby in a clean bottle. Concentrated liquid formula is more expensive than powdered. To use ready-to-feed formula, just open and pour into a clean baby bottle.

Standard Formulas

Parents most often pick a cow's-milk–based formula to nourish their infants. And with good reason. Most children thrive on a cow's-milk formula fortified with iron. Milk-based formulas are available with little iron, or as iron-fortified, but only iron-fortified formula meets an infant's needs for this vital nutrient.

Manufacturers remove the butterfat from milk, replacing it with vegetable oil or a mixture of vegetable and animal fats. Changing the fat composition improves the digestibility and increases the concentration of essential fats needed to foster peak growth and development.

Common Brand Names: Good Start (Carnation); Enfamil with Iron and Enfamil Low Iron (Mead Johnson); and Similac with Iron (Ross)

Soy Formulas

There are very few medical reasons why a baby would need soy formula, yet sales account for about 25 percent of the infant formula market. Obviously, parents see soy formulas as either beneficial or necessary, or both.

All soy formulas contain the necessary added iron and meet the requirements for vitamins and minerals set by the AAP and the FDA. They do not contain lactose. When comparing labels of cow's-milk formula and that of soy, don't be surprised to see higher levels of protein, calcium, and phosphorus. Soy formulas need more of these nutrients because they are not absorbed as well by the body as when they are found in cow's-milk formulas.

Soy-based formulas are just as nutritious for full-term, healthy infants as formulas made from cow's milk, but experts aren't so sure that premature babies should consume soy formula. If your baby was born before term, ask your doctor about using soy formulas.

When does a soy-based formula make sense? If you have a baby:

- With galactosemia, an inborn error of metabolism that prohibits him from breaking down the carbohydrate in milk and milk products;
- Who is lactose intolerant and cannot fully digest lactose, the primary carbohydrate in cow's milk;
- Who you want to raise as a strict vegetarian;
- Who is recovering from an intestinal infection.

Many parents switch their babies to soy formula because they are convinced that their baby's abdominal discomfort or allergy symptoms from drinking a cow's-milk–based formula will disappear. Yet, about half of all infants who are allergic to cow's-milk protein cannot tolerate soy protein, either. Before switching to soy, ask you pediatrician. If your child is allergic to milk and to soy, he may need a protein hydrosolate formula.

Common Brand Names: Alsoy (Carnation); Isomil (Ross); ProSoBee (Mead Johnson)

Lactose-Free Formulas

These cow's-milk–based formulas come free of lactose. Infants who cannot digest lactose, the carbohydrate in cow's milk, can still drink lactose-free cow's-milk formula.

Common Brand Names: Enfamil LactoFree (Mead Johnson); Similac Lactose Free Infant Formula (Ross)

Protein Hydrosolate Formulas

Lactose-free protein hydrosolate formulas contain protein that is broken down to prevent an allergic response. This type of formula may be attractive to parents of colicky babies and those with a suspected intolerance to lactose, the primary carbohydrate in milk.

Protein hydrosolates work well in babies that are allergic to both cow's-milk protein and soy protein, and for infants with certain conditions that hamper the proper digestion and absorption of nutrients, including cystic fibrosis and intestinal surgery. While protein hydrosolate formulas are costlier than cow- or soy-based options, they are a cheaper, less invasive alternative to feeding babies through a major artery.

Common Brand Names: Alimentum (Ross), Nutramigen (Mead Johnson), Pregestimil (Mead Johnson)

Follow-Up Formula

Your baby can begin taking follow-up formulas at six months as long as he's eating solid foods and growing normally. But are follow-up formulas *necessary?* No. Will follow-up formulas hurt your child? Another no. You can continue to decrease the amount of regular formula and increase solid foods until your child reaches the age of one. At a year, he or she can start drinking whole milk instead of formula.

Common Brand Names: Follow-Up (Carnation), Follow-Up Soy (Carnation)

When Milk Is Not the Beverage of Choice

Any type of formula is more expensive than breastfeeding. It's also costlier than regular cow's, goat's, canned condensed, and evaporated milk. But giving any type of milk to infants in place of commercial formula could cost your child in the long run.

Milk is not an option for any baby under the age of one, says the AAP. Milk cannot supply the nutrients babies need to thrive. For one, milk is low in iron. Using milk of any type instead of breast milk or iron-fortified formula promotes iron deficiency, which hampers brain development. To make matters worse, babies can be sensitive to the protein in milk (infants with milk allergies are often sensitive to soy as well), resulting in chronic blood loss from the intestinal tract. Bleeding is the primary route for iron loss from the body, so everyday blood loss further exacerbates an infant's low iron stores.

There are other reasons for babies to avoid milk. When infants drink milk in place of formula or breast milk, they risk consuming excess sodium, potassium, and chloride, which can strain their kidneys. Milk is also deficient in the type of fat that best fosters brain development, as well as vitamin E and zinc. What's more, infants fed reduced-fat milk risk consuming too much protein and inadequate calories and fat to fuel their growth.

PREPARING AND HANDLING INFANT FORMULA

Babies have delicate systems that are in a state of flux. That's why you should minimize the potential for troublesome germs when preparing baby's formula.

When preparing to feed baby any type of formula, begin by washing your hands with warm soapy water for at least twenty seconds, making sure to clean thoroughly under your nails. Dry hands with a clean towel.

Bottles and Nipples

Regardless of which kind of formula you choose, you must have clean feeding equipment or risk intestinal illness. After washing with warm, soapy water and rinsing thoroughly, boil bottles and nipples in a large covered pot for at least five minutes and not more than ten to make sure they are germ free. You can use a dishwasher that supplies heated water and has a hot drying cycle to clean baby bottles, but I have found that nipples must be boiled in order for them to come completely clean.

Water Supply

Cover and boil tap or bottled water for at least five minutes to reduce the chance of bacterial contamination that could make baby sick. Cool the water for at least fifteen minutes to make it easier and safer to mix with formula. Make sure to keep a lid on the water so that it remains sterile.

There are a couple of things to think about when weighing your options for the water used to make your child's formula. First and foremost, lead. Infants and children who consume lead risk long-term growth problems and learning disabilities, as this toxic metal wreaks havoc on brain development. Your home, apartment, or condominium may have lead pipes, particularly if it was constructed before 1986. Even newer dwellings using copper pipes to transport water are not completely safe, since the pipes could be connected with lead solder. Lead leaches into tap water and can make its way into infant formula (see "Get the Lead Out," page 60, for how to determine if your drinking water contains lead).

Fluoride is a mineral that your water may lack. Most likely, the water coming into your home contains added fluoride, which is critical for strong teeth and bones. As long as it's lead-free, tap water is acceptable for making formula. If you prefer bottled water, you could be shortchanging your child when it comes to fluoride. That's because bottled waters are not required to contain fluoride. If you're unsure whether the bottled water you give to your child contains fluoride, here's what to do:

- Call the number on the label to find out the fluoride content.
- If there's no number to call, switch to another brand that can supply the information you need.
- Ask your pediatrician if the fluoride level in your bottled water is sufficient for your child.

Formula

Wipe clean the top of the infant formula can to remove dust and dirt that may fall into the formula as you open the container. Make sure measuring spoons and cups are clean.

You can save time by mixing up a day's worth of formula at a time in a large container, then pouring it into individual bottles. Or store formula in a quart-size container and pour into baby bottles as needed for feedings.

Always prepare concentrated liquid formula and powdered formula according to the manufacturer's directions on the label. Using less than the recommended amount of formula means baby will not receive adequate calories and nutrients for growth and development. There's no reason to add more formula to the mix or to use less water unless your pediatrician advises it. Additional formula won't make your child any smarter, stronger, or taller, but it can endanger his health. Excess formula can burden a child's kidneys and cause other serious disorders, including dehydration.

Never add solids such as infant cereal or any other substance, including medication and any form of sugar, to an infant's bottle for any reason.

Handling It

Always immediately refrigerate any open cans of ready-to-feed formula and any mixture of concentrated liquid or powdered formula and water.

Mixed formula is good for forty-eight hours as long as it is properly refrigerated, the bottles are clean and properly sealed, and your refrigerator thermometer registers no higher than 39°F. After forty-eight hours, discard any unused formula. Likewise, pitch what's left over in the bottle when baby doesn't finish the entire amount.

Never refrigerate leftover breast milk or infant formula from a previous feeding to give to your baby later on. As baby sucks, the bacteria from her mouth can get into the bottle and multiply, causing intestinal illness should you use the leftover milk.

Focus on Safe Formula

Parents don't always prepare and handle formula the way they should, despite having read, and claiming to understand, manufacturers' directions. According to a study in the *Journal of the American Dietetic Association*, researchers found that 33 percent of moms mixed formula with warm water directly out of the tap (cooled boiled water is recommended) and nearly half of the mothers heated baby bottles in a microwave (frowned upon because of the risk of burns). In addition, when infant formula was left at room temperature for more than two hours (it should be refrigerated at all times), the chances for diarrhea in older infants increased. Other potentially harmful practices included diluting formula, putting baby to bed with a bottle, and adding cereal or medicine to prepared formula.

Feeding the Baby

There's no scientific proof that babies prefer warm formula, but it's fine to serve it that way. Resist the temptation to microwave bottles of formula for speedy warm-up, however. Microwaving infant formula can be harmful. Microwave heating is uneven, making it difficult to monitor the temperature of the formula in the bottle's center. The bottle may feel only slightly warm, but steam can build within the bottle, causing an explosion and spraying hot milk that can badly burn an infant.

Always cradle your baby in a semiupright position in the crook of your arm when feeding, and tilt her bottle so that the nipple fills with milk. Never prop up a bottle for your daughter to feed from. It's a health risk, and it's antisocial. Feeding your baby is an opportunity for you to spend some quiet time holding and speaking to her, and a chance for her to study your face and get to know it, as well as to listen to your voice.

Begin feeding by gently brushing baby on one cheek with your finger or with the nipple of the bottle, so that she will instinctively turn toward the bottle while opening her mouth. Once her mouth is open, slide the nipple nearly all the way in, but gently. Your baby should begin to suck immediately, but it could take a few tries, so repeat the process as often as necessary, and try not to get frustrated!

Bottle-fed babies, be it formula or breast milk, typically need to burp more than babies who get milk from the breast. That's because infants take in more air as they suck from a bottle. If your baby begins to snooze after a feeding, let her be. If not, try gently burping her. Burping can make way for more formula in the stomach, so that you can feed her until she is full. Never force a bottle on an infant.

HOW MUCH IS ENOUGH AND HOW OFTEN TO FEED

Like breastfed babies, infants nourished with formula should be allowed to feed on demand. That helps them to eat only when they are hungry, which sets the stage for easier weight control in the future.

Babies sleep a lot just after birth. During the first few days of his life, your baby will take very little at a sitting, perhaps just an ounce or two, but he will need to eat frequently (see the chart with suggested number of bottle feedings on page 92). Don't allow sleeping babies to miss a feeding because you don't want to wake them, or think that you should not. Wake baby after three hours and offer him a bottle to ward off the risk of dehydration and malnutrition.

Your baby's appetite kicks in soon enough and his formula consumption should, and typically does, increase accordingly. Infants need to drink enough formula to put on about one ounce of weight every day during the first three months. Your regular visit to the pediatrician during this time will help the doctor gauge your baby's development. Growth slows to about a half ounce gain a day between three and six months, and babies gain even less than that as they get closer to their first birthday.

Don't feel badly when your newborn doesn't drink the whole bottle or eat according to the suggested intakes below. Babies should be fed when they are hungry. Parents must recognize and respect their child's signals that they are full and not try to overfeed them to comply with arbitrary eating goals.

Like their breastfed counterparts, formula-fed babies do not require extra fluid unless it is very hot and humid outside.

Suggested Number and Volume of Bottle Feedings for a Normal Infant

Age	Number of Daily Bottles	Amount of Formula in Each Bottle
Birth to 1 week	6 to 10	1 to 3 ounces
1 week to 1 month	7 to 8	2 to 4 ounces
1 month to 3 months	5 to 7	4 to 6 ounces
3 months to 6 months*	4 to 5	6 to 7 ounces
6 months to 9 months	3 to 4	7 to 8 ounces
10 months to 12 months	3	7 to 8 ounces

*You can begin feeding your child solid foods such as iron-fortified infant cereal at four months of age. Formula consumption tends to begin declining after six months because it's assumed that your baby will be eating more solid foods as time goes on.

Source: Manual of Pediatric Nutrition, D. G. Kelts and E. G. Jones. (Boston: Little Brown and Company, 1984), p. 38.

COLIC

Every baby cries for no obvious reason at some point. You may put down persistent crying to simple gas, but if you child's crying jags persist day after day and start in late afternoon or evening, then colic is probably culpable.

Colic is characterized by inconsolable wailing (and sometimes shrieking) that begins around two to six weeks of age. Crying jags seem to come out of nowhere and to last forever. No one is sure of colic's cause, but it appears that abdominal discomfort is at the root of the crying that severely taxes everyone's nerves. Of course, your child could be crying because of another medical condition, which is why you should speak with your pediatrician.

Formula-fed infants are more vulnerable to colic than are breastfed babies. A colicky baby could be allergic to cow's-milk-based formula, but don't switch her over to soy without your pediatrician's approval: Babies who are allergic to the protein in cow's milk may be equally sensitive to soy protein. Your colicky infant may fare well with a formula containing predigested protein, which helps avoid triggering an allergic reaction.

Heading Off Feeding Problems

Most babies can polish off a bottle in about fifteen to twenty minutes. Newborns may need some time to become accustomed to the nipple, so feedings may go more slowly. As long as your baby seems satisfied with a feeding, she is drinking about as much as recommended in the chart on page 92, and her pediatrician says her growth is on target, then things are probably going well.

Sometimes it takes infants more than twenty minutes to finish a bottle. When this happens consistently, call your pediatrician, since your baby may need to be evaluated for motor delay problems that limit his ability to suck properly on the nipple. But baby's feeding problem may have little to do with his physical prowess. When the hole in the plastic nipple is too small, babies must work much harder to get the formula out. They can get tuckered out from the effort and stop feeding well before they are satiated. Perhaps the nipple collapses during feeding, or it's clogged. If you suspect clogging, test the flow of formula by tipping the bottle upside down. The fluid should drip out under pressure. Some infants suck in a lot of air during bottle-feeding, which limits their stomach capacity. Try gently burping baby midway through each feeding to maximize nourishment.

When nursing infants are colicky, some dietary changes may be in order on mom's part. Breastfed babies could be hypersensitive to cow's-milk protein, which can make its way into an infant's digestive tract intact through breast milk. Some babies seem to feel better when their mothers avoid milk products, peanuts, eggs, seafood, and wheat, particularly when allergies run in the family. Food avoidance does not always solve the problem, however. Even so, eliminating gas-producing foods such as cabbage, broccoli, and cauliflower may help, too.

Colic does go away, usually by the time a child is four months old. While you're waiting for colic to disappear, there are a few strategies for preserving your sanity and calming your baby. Experts say colicky babies should avoid unnecessary stimulation. Some parents swear by rocking a wailing baby or taking him for a walk or a car ride, as babies seem to be soothed by rhythmic motions. Ask your pediatrician if medication is a possibility, too.

Chapter 5

From Four Months to One Year

Each time I feed him the
first spoonful of food
at a meal, he makes a
face like it's disgusting,
even though he's had it
plenty of times.

—Hillary, *mother of three boys*

WHAT'S HAPPENING NOW: DEVELOPMENTAL MILESTONES

Babies change a lot between four and twelve months. During this critical period of growth, an infant's physical development not only affects what they eat, but how. In eight months, infants go from total dependence on breast milk or formula to consuming finger foods and drinking from a sippy cup while sitting up.

By the time she reaches her first birthday, your child will have the majority of her primary teeth. Her muscles will be stronger, and she will have gained greater control over them. She will be thrilled by what she can do with her body. You will witness your child's joy as she learns to roll over at about six months; moves on to crawling a few months later, and perhaps walking before the age of one; and when she grabs objects, including food, and attempts to get them into her mouth.

Brain development continues at a frenzied pace, and nutrition plays a huge role. A baby's babbling and cooing are important signs of language development that you should take seriously. Your child's gurgles and grunts are his attempt to communicate with you. Looking directly at your baby when talking to him, particularly at mealtimes, is a source of pleasure and provides positive stimulation that promotes cognition. Plus, conversing with baby goes a long way toward enhancing his language skills. Experts say babies understand what you are saying to them well before they can verbalize their own thoughts.

One of the most noteworthy nutritional milestones of a child's life occurs between four and six months of age. That's when you may first safely feed your child solid foods. Before four months, your baby's intestinal tract has not matured enough to handle the likes of infant cereal and pureed vegetables. Introducing foods before the recommended time raises the risk of food allergies. This is particularly true of children born to highly allergic families, even though food allergies are relatively uncommon. See more about food allergies in Chapter 12.

Most children are developmentally ready to begin eating some solid food by six months of age. Your baby must be capable of supporting his own head to consume solids, even if he is not ready to sit up on his own. By about four to five months, babies no longer have the extrusion reflex, which is the natural urge to push anything but liquid from the mouth, so they are more accepting of a spoon. Also, between four and six months is when an infant's swallowing has improved to the point where he can handle semisolid foods such as fortified infant cereal, preferably mixed with formula or breast milk.

At six to eight months of age, most babies have begun mastering the pincer grasp, which develops when they use the muscles of their thumb and forefinger to pick up small objects. Providing safe finger foods during this time helps children strengthen their grasping skills and then to move on to actually getting the food into their mouth, which often occurs at seven to nine months.

In My Experience
There's No Rush for Solid Foods

Your child is four months old and you're eager to feed him cereal so he'll be bigger, stronger, or smarter. Relax. As long as you begin food between four and six months of age, you're doing fine by your baby. Hayley, my oldest, began eating iron-fortified infant cereal around four and a half months, but Hannah didn't begin until around the five-and-a-half-month mark. At the time each child began infant cereal, she was on a steady diet of a combination of breast milk and formula, so I knew that she was getting the necessary nutrition. Remember, each baby is different. Some children are simply more interested in eating than others. For others, taking nourishment from a spoon is so foreign that they need more time to accept the idea. Don't wait too long, however. Experts say that going much beyond six months before trying to get infants to accept solid foods makes it more difficult. Plus, it's nutritionally risky.

STARTING SOLIDS

Parents often tell me that once they got the hang of it, learning to feed a newborn was a relative breeze compared to introducing solids to an older infant. I agree. As someone who has been through the transition three times, I know that it is rarely smooth and certainly not predictable.

The security and ease of nourishing your child with breast milk or infant formula vanishes when solids enter the picture, particularly when babies develop teeth (and begin biting you during nursing) or become distracted by what's going on around them when you're giving them a bottle. Then there's the uncertainty of each meal: Will she eat? How much cereal should she eat? Will she like this or that new fruit or vegetable? And how long should I try to get her to accept food at any meal before giving up?

When you worry about your infant's opposition to solid foods, or think that your baby is not eating enough, you can end up stressed at mealtime. This is especially true when you're trying to simultaneously monitor other children and eat your own meal. Alleviate some of the tension by arming yourself with a few simple facts and tips about introducing solid foods into baby's diet.

Satisfy calorie needs. Until baby reaches six months, he requires about 650 calories a day; from six to twelve months, about 850 will suffice. Even if your infant begins solids at four months, chances are breast milk or infant formula will continue to supply the majority of his energy until at least six months. By the time he reaches twelve months, he should be taking in more than half of his calories as table food.

Keep it relaxed. Feeding a well-rested baby who is hungry but not ravenous is easier and more rewarding that trying to feed a cranky or tired one. Your child should be interested in eating, not irritated by it.

Sit her up. Your baby must be able to hold up her head to be ready to receive solids. Sit your baby upright in an infant seat or prop her in a highchair supported by towels.

Feed baby first. Whenever the baby ate before the rest of the family, I had more time to spend with her without worrying about what the other kids were eating during the meal. Of course, time (and baby's hunger level) does not always permit this type of one-on-one feeding. But I recommend it when you are starting solids with your baby and you have older children, because it relieves some of the pressure, reduces distractions, and keeps baby and you more relaxed. When you're not constantly jumping up from the table to get a family member a fork or a glass of milk, or to wipe up a spill (as Tom and I are), you have more time to talk with your baby about the food she's eating or about anything else you please, you can better assess her hunger level, and you can pay attention to the cues she's giving you about what and how much she wants to eat. As time goes on and your baby eats more consistently at meals, it will become easier to feed her with the rest of the family. Even when she eats before or after the family meal, always seat her at the table with you for the social interaction.

Make it nutritious. Begin your foray into solid foods with fortified rice cereal mixed with formula or breast milk. Mix about one teaspoon dry infant cereal with four or so teaspoons of breast milk or (premixed) infant formula for each feeding.

It's not written in stone that baby's first solid food must be rice cereal, but it's surely a sound idea. Although most types of baby cereals are fortified with iron and other important minerals and vitamins, rice cereal is gluten-free, making it a safer alternative. Gluten is the part of wheat that can cause allergies in some people.

Why not try pureed vegetables or fruit before cereal? Because they lack the iron baby needs for good health. By six months of age, an infant's body has gone through much of his iron stores, which is why he requires additional daily iron from foods.

Keep it varied. Once baby becomes accustomed to infant cereal, move on to pureed fruits and vegetables (see "Infant Feeding Guide," page 105). Serving baby a variety of foods encourages a healthier diet from the get-go. Expand your child's eating horizons by encouraging her to try foods you don't normally eat because you dislike them.

Serve up small portions. Initially, your baby won't recognize solid foods as nourishment, so don't expect him to polish off a bowl of baby food during the first few weeks of eating solid foods. More than likely, your child will take just a small amount of food at each meal, at least to begin with. As infants become increasingly familiar with eating solids, they readily open their mouths to take larger bites.

Breastfeeding Makes for Vegetable Eaters

According to a study in *Pediatrics*, breastfed infants may be more likely to eat vegetables between four and six months. Why? It's possible that because breast milk provides exposure to a variety of flavors, children have a broader, and more accepting, palate. The study also provided breastfed and formula-fed infants the same food ten different times and found that after the tenth time, consumption went up in both groups. Breastfed infants ate more of the vegetables, however.

One at a time. Introduce single ingredient foods, such as rice cereal, instead of a blend of baby cereal grains and do it one at a time. Feed just one new food to your child for five days or so before adding others. Why wait? It's your chance to see whether your baby has trouble tolerating a particular food. When you add too many foods at once, it's harder to pinpoint food allergies or other sensitivities should they occur. For example, once your baby has tried the different types of cereal grains without incident, then you may use a mixed grain infant cereal with confidence. Look for baby foods marketed as "First Foods" as they tend to contain just one ingredient. Even so, it may be difficult to tell which foods contain single ingredients, so read the ingredient label carefully. As your child matures, he can move on to mixtures such as tropical fruit blends, but he should avoid toddler foods until about a year. Toddler foods may contain chunks of food that could result in choking.

Come back to it. My kids would give me a "What's this?" face each time I put the spoon in their mouth at a meal, even when they had eaten the food before. Don't be daunted. It doesn't mean your child isn't hungry or that she won't eat. Babies often spit out the first bit of food you give them at each meal, as if they are getting adjusted to eating from a spoon all over again. This reaction gradually disappears as eating utensils become a regular part of their meals. Your baby may reject a food the first time you offer it, but accept it days, weeks, or months later. That could mean he's trying to adjust to a new taste or texture. Try serving a new food with an old favorite to increase acceptance, and don't give up!

Food Allergy Red Flags

Will your child be allergic to food? You won't know until you try feeding him. Food allergy symptoms can make themselves known within minutes or up to a few hours after eating a food for the second time. Always alert your pediatrician if any of the following signs of food allergy appears:

- Abdominal pain
- Diarrhea
- Dry or raspy cough
- Excessive crankiness
- Excessive gas
- Hives
- Itching and/or tightness in the throat
- Itchy eyes
- Nausea
- Rash (eczema)
- Runny nose
- Shortness of breath
- Stomach bloating
- Vomiting
- Wheezing

Don't force it. A baby's appetite varies, so stay tuned to your child's hunger cues. When an infant doesn't feel in tip-top shape because of teething, fever, nasal congestion, or an ear infection, she'll eat less. Once she's feeling better, her appetite should pick up. When a child turns his head away as you try to feed him, it probably means he's not interested in taking food from you. Children are not always hungry when their parents are, and they may not eat according to the clock. Whatever the case, stay calm. Caregivers who try to feed unwilling infants make children tense and more likely to refuse food the next time around. That can set off a vicious cycle where baby senses your anxiety and perhaps anger and continues to brush off food. As you relax about feeding him, he relaxes, too. Surely, every parent gets frustrated from time to time. But if you are having trouble at every meal, speak to your pediatrician to get help.

Don't be a clean freak. You child will dribble mashed fruit down her chin, plunge her tiny mitts into a bowl of cereal and smear it on her face, and methodically toss food to the floor, just to see it fall. Be prepared for a mess, but don't worry about it. Order is not your first priority as a parent trying to foster acceptance of a well-balanced diet. Wiping your child's face and hands after every bite can turn him into a fretful being who becomes too concerned with your reaction to his messiness to try out his eating skills.

In My Experience
Babies Don't Need Fruit Juice

Parents perceive juice as healthy, and, in general, it is. Depending on the brand, 100 percent fruit juice products can be rich in calcium, vitamin C, and disease-fighting phytochemicals, substances exclusive to plant foods. But is juice necessary for infants? The answer is no. In fact, juice can be quite detrimental, especially when it replaces milk in a baby's bottle. While juice provides calories, vitamins, and minerals, it should never pinch-hit for the more nutritious fortified infant formula or for breast milk, which contains the nutrients babies require to flourish. Substituting juice for milk may stunt a child's growth. And infants allowed to suck on a bottle full of any carbohydrate-rich fluid such as juice or milk for prolonged periods risk baby bottle tooth decay. That's because the bacteria in the baby's mouth uses the constant supply of carbohydrate coming out of the bottle as an energy source to produce acid that rots tooth enamel. Letting a baby repeatedly fall asleep with a baby bottle full of juice in his mouth is problematic for this reason. I have never filled up a baby bottle with juice and fed it to any of my girls, and I don't recommend you do, either. When children are ready to use a sippy cup, then they can have fruit juice, but no more than six ounces a day, and preferably less. It's OK, but not required, to mix fortified 100 percent fruit juice with infant cereals beginning at four months, as long as you don't serve baby orange, grapefruit, or tomato juice. And forget about special juices designed for babies. They are expensive, and they are no better for your child. In fact, "baby" juices can cost upwards of two and a half times more than regular juice.

For safety's sake. Never leave children unattended when eating. Don't allow older kids to feed the baby without you around, either. Older children can be overzealous when feeding little ones, causing choking.

Unless you intend to use the entire amount of baby food or throw away the remainder, don't feed an infant directly from a baby food jar. The bacteria from baby's mouth gets into the food, multiplies, and can cause illness when you feed the leftovers to her later on. Instead, spoon some food into a separate dish and refrigerate the rest. If you go back to get more food from the same jar, use a clean spoon, not the one you are using to feed baby during the meal.

BABY FOOD: TO BUY OR TO MAKE?

Homemade or store-bought? For some parents, the decision is easy: stock up on small jars of pureed fruits, vegetables, and meats. Others opt to do it themselves, preparing baby food at home. Even though time is spent in planning and preparation, homemade baby food cuts costs. But homemade foods for baby aren't necessarily nutritionally superior. For example, all ready-to-eat baby fruits in jars are fortified with vitamin C; there is little produce suitable for babies that can boast similar levels in its natural state.

No matter which route you take, you must purchase the iron-fortified infant cereal that is an integral part of your baby's diet.

Make-It-Yourself Baby Food: The Basics

- Thoroughly wash fresh produce, and remove peels, cores, and seeds. Follow strict food safety rules for preparing and storing homemade baby foods. (See Chapter 11 for more on food safety.)
- Bake, broil, or stew meats. Remove the skin before serving meat and trim all visible fat. Puree in blender to desired consistency with a small amount of fluid. For older infants, chop meat and poultry into very small pieces.
- Whenever possible, use fresh fruits and vegetables, and cook with very little water to best preserve nutrition. Don't leave produce lying around in the refrigerator for too long, either. Cook within a few days for maximum nutrition.
- Avoid using canned fruits and vegetables with added salt or sugar.
- Have on hand a food processor or food mill for the purpose of pureeing or mashing foods.
- Never add honey to an infant's food. Honey can cause botulism, a food-borne illness that's dangerous for babies.
- Serve plain foods. Reserve a portion of food for your infant and then add salt, pepper, and other seasonings you desire for the rest of the family to eat.
- Use homemade refrigerated food within forty-eight hours after preparing.
- When preparing pureed food in batches, freeze some in ice cube trays and

cover well for later use. Label and date all containers. Always thaw the desired amount in the refrigerator, never on the kitchen countertop.

- Never feed your baby homemade pureed beets, turnips, collard greens, or spinach. They contain naturally occurring nitrates that can result in anemia. Ready-to-eat baby food versions of these vegetables are safe because food manufacturers test for nitrates.
- Avoid adding raw or cooked egg whites to baby's food. Egg whites may cause an allergic reaction in children under the age of one, and raw egg whites are a food-borne illness risk.

Storing Baby Food: What to Keep, When to Pitch

Label baby foods to ensure their safety. No date on your child's food? When in doubt, throw it out. Otherwise, follow this advice from the USDA about how long you may safely keep baby foods on hand.

Opened or Freshly Made	Lasts in the Refrigerator For	Lasts in the Freezer For
Strained fruits and vegetables	2–3 days	6–8 months
Strained meats and eggs	1 day	1–2 months
Meat/vegetable combinations	1–2 days	1–2 months

Commercial Baby Food: Best Buys

Store-bought baby foods are ready to eat, plentiful, and relatively fuss free—a plus for busy parents on the go. Choices abound in the baby food aisle, the biggest one being whether to go with organic brands. Organic food has grown in popularity with adults, many of whom desire the same for their babies. Organic baby foods such as Gerber's Organic Harvest and Earth's Best are costlier than their mainstream counterparts, largely because the organic foods industry is not as cost-efficient.

In making a decision about using organic foods, it helps to know what the certified organic label means. Put simply, organic baby foods contain plant foods grown without synthetic chemicals. The animal products used in organic baby foods have been produced without antibiotics or added hormones. Organic ingredients are free of preservatives, dyes, and waxes, too.

Whether purchasing organic baby food or the mainstream variety, always steer clear of products with added salt or sugar, including corn syrup and modified starch, as they tend to be needless fillers.

INFANT FEEDING GUIDE

It's not always easy to know what to feed a growing infant. Here are some guidelines to help you month by month. Each stage builds upon the last. The amounts listed here are averages. Don't worry if your baby is eating more or less than the suggested amounts as long as your pediatrician says he is growing properly.

Note: If allergies run in your family, you must delay the introduction of certain foods to baby. Read "Food Allergy and Intolerance," Chapter 12, for more information before you begin feeding baby solid foods.

Age: 4–6 Months
- Breast milk: Feed on demand, usually about 4–7 times daily, or
- Iron-fortified infant formula: 24–40 ounces daily, or more as needed
- Iron-fortified infant cereal: Mix 2–3 teaspoons rice cereal (to begin with) or barley cereal with formula, water, or breast milk to create a semisolid consistency. Offer twice a day. Don't expect baby to eat much at first.
- Fruit and fruit juices: None needed, but you may mix 100 percent fruit juice with infant cereal in place of formula or breast milk. Avoid citrus and tomato juices for now. It's OK to offer small amounts of pureed fruits to baby now, too.

Age: 6–8 Months
- Breast milk: Feed on demand, usually about 4–5 times daily, or
- Iron-fortified infant formula: 24–32 ounces daily
- Iron-fortified infant cereals: Mix 3–9 tablespoons infant cereal with formula, water, or breast milk in two or more feedings daily
- Fruit and fruit juices: Pureed, strained, or mashed fruits, such as bananas and applesauce: 1 jar or ½ cup a day, split into 2–3 feedings. Offer fruit instead of fruit juice.
- Vegetables: Strained or mashed, cooked vegetables. Dark yellow, dark green, or orange, but no corn. Start with mild-tasting vegetables such as green beans, peas, or squash. Give ½ to 1 jar baby food vegetables, or ¼ to ½ cup per day.

Age: 8–10 Months
- Breast milk: Feed on demand, usually about 3–4 feedings daily, or
- Iron-fortified infant formula: 16–32 ounces daily
- Iron-fortified infant cereals, or plain hot cereals: About ¼ to ½ cup a day, but this will vary.

Breads: Toast, bagel, or crackers for teething, if desired. Always supervise baby.

- Fruit and fruit juices: OK to serve citrus and tomato juice now, but don't let juice replace fruit. Baby can have 1–2 jars of pureed fruit a day, or finely chopped, peeled soft fruit wedges, including bananas, peaches, pears, and apples.
- Vegetables: 1–2 jars of pureed vegetables or ½ to 1 cup daily.
- Protein foods: Begin offering fresh ground or finely chopped chicken or lean meats with all the bones, fat, and skin removed; full-fat yogurt; hard cheeses such as cheddar; mashed cooked dried beans; cooked egg yolks; and peanut butter thinned with applesauce or full-fat yogurt.

Age: 10–12 Months
- Breast milk: Feed on demand, usually 3–4 feedings daily, or
- Iron-fortified infant formula: 16–24 ounces daily
- Milk: Full-fat milk can be offered, beginning at *one year*. Make the transition by mixing formula with some milk and gradually increasing the amount of milk, until milk completely replaces formula.
- Cereals and breads: Infant or cooked cereals, bread, mashed potatoes, rice, and pasta, a tablespoon or so at a time. Intake will vary.
- Vegetables: Cooked vegetables. Some raw vegetables as tolerated by child.
- Fruit and fruit juices: All fresh fruits, peeled and seeded, or canned fruits are OK for baby now. Just make sure they are soft and cut into small pieces.
- Protein foods: Small pieces of fresh chopped chicken, lean meat, or fish with all the bones, fat, and skin removed; full-fat yogurt, cottage cheese, and cheese; mashed cooked dried beans; cooked *whole* eggs beginning at twelve months; and peanut butter thinned with applesauce or full-fat yogurt.

IMPORTANT FIRST-YEAR FEEDING TIPS
- Use baby spoon to feed baby solid foods. Do not put infant cereal in bottles filled with formula or breast milk. This practice encourages overfeeding.
- Do not give cow's milk or fortified soy milk to baby until her first birthday. Provide full-fat milk until she reaches her second birthday.
- Introduce one food at a time. Wait five days between new foods.
- Never put your baby to bed with a bottle because it increases the risk of tooth decay.

Chapter 6

From One to

Three Years

Samantha is so set in her eating
that she screams and snarls at
us when we try to give her new
foods. You'd think we were
offering her mud, or worse!
Every once in a while, she'll
cave in and give a new food
a try, which is rewarding,
since she usually likes it.

—Winnie, mother of a two-year-old and an infant

WHAT'S HAPPENING NOW: DEVELOPMENTAL MILESTONES

You may think of him as such, but your child is no longer a baby in the strict sense of the word. He's a toddler now, and the name fits kids ages one through three. Talk about rough and tumble! Once standing becomes old hat, toddlers try their luck at walking, and have their share of spills. Making your way around the room with feet planted wide apart for support is never smooth sailing.

Before you know it, walking is a breeze for your daughter. After they are up and about, children are much more physically active than they were as infants. At this point in her life, your child seems to possess endless energy reserves, even though her appetite appears to have taken a nosedive from her days as a baby. What gives? Infants grow at a frantic pace during year one. In fact, there's no other time when children grow faster. But a child's growth slows considerably after her first birthday. Despite a toddler's frenetic pace, she actually requires fewer calories per pound.

She may not be packing on the pounds or getting taller before your eyes, but your toddler's brain development hasn't slowed one iota. It seems that healthy toddlers learn new ways to communicate every day. For sure, youngest toddlers use more garbled words, grunts, and body language to get their message across. But as her third birthday approaches, a youngster's vocabulary has usually developed by leaps and bounds. That's when she begins to string together words in short sentences and ask a lot of questions, allowing her personality to shine through. Despite their burgeoning vocabulary, one- and two-year-olds often lack the words to completely express their emotions, which may result in temper tantrums thrown out of frustration, including at mealtimes.

Loving, sociable beings one minute; screaming and out of control the next. That's the lot of many toddlers, who are studies in contradiction.

For instance, toddlers love routine. The daily rituals played out in your household and at day care send the signal that everything is OK in their world. Older toddlers take particular comfort in knowing what will happen next. Yet, one- and two-year-olds tend to rebel against highly structured activities. Why? Their short attention span and natural curiosity about their environment makes them easily distracted.

A toddler's unpredictability can be particularly exasperating for parents during mealtimes. When you're one or two years old, your appetite changes from day to day, making it hard for parents to gauge what and how much food to prepare and offer. Periodic growth spurts result in a greater demand for food over a very short time, since kids can add an inch to their frames in a matter of days. Likewise, teething (most often molars), colds, and ear infections can dampen your son's desire for food. During this stage, your child will also begin to want to feed himself as well as let you know what he would like to eat.

The addition of cow's milk to your child's diet is a dietary milestone. After he reaches a year, you may substitute cow's milk or fortified soy beverages for breast milk or formula. If you are nursing, you can continue for as long as you and your baby desire, but be aware that solid foods should dominate the diet by one year of age.

Make It Milk

The risk of food allergy is greatly reduced by age one. That's why it's safe to give your child full-fat cow's milk or fortified soy beverage instead of infant formula or breast milk. Here's how to make a safe and effective transition to milk or a soy beverage.

- Replace a quarter of the formula or expressed breast milk with full-fat cow's milk or soy beverage and gradually increase the proportion over the course of a couple of weeks or so.
- Provide about 16 to 24 ounces of milk or soy beverage a day to a one- or two-year-old to help ensure adequate protein and calcium intake.
- Use only full-fat milk until age two. Full-fat milk provides the necessary fat and calories for your child's growth and cholesterol for his brain development. Children can begin drinking reduced-fat varieties such as 2% reduced-fat milk or 1% low-fat milk at age two, but it may not be necessary to serve lower fat milks. When milk, full-fat fortified soy beverages, and other dairy products are a major part of a child's diet, using reduced-fat versions can hamper growth by restricting fat, a concentrated calorie source.

EXPANDING YOUR CHILD'S DIET

Even though he's only one or two years old, it's never too early to help a child begin to develop healthy eating habits. You can do this in part by offering a variety of nutritious foods that are appropriate for your child's developmental stage. For the most part, you can put away the baby food now. After age one, your child can eat just about anything, as long as he's not allergic to it, and as long as it's in kid-friendly form—either pureed, mashed, or cut into small pieces.

It's one thing to prepare and serve healthy foods. What's tough is figuring out whether you're feeding a child the right amount. How do you know how much to serve?

The Pyramid Plan on page 43 is based on the USDA Food Guide Pyramid for Young Children, which applies to kids age two and up. It provides the details about what and how much your two-year-old should eat.

One-year-olds are another matter. You could go by the "rule of one," as I call it: Serve one tablespoon of each food you're eating at a meal for each year of your child's life, plus the recommended 16 to 24 ounces of milk throughout the day. So, if you're having mashed potatoes, steamed carrots, and chicken for dinner, serve a one-year-old at least a tablespoon of each food.

Here's a suggested daily feeding guide for a one-year-old.

Breakfast
   4 ounces whole milk
   ¼ cup whole grain ready-to-eat cereal
   ¼ medium banana

Snack
   2 graham cracker squares
   4 ounces 100 percent juice, preferably fortified with
      vitamin C and/or calcium

Lunch
   4 ounces whole milk
   1 ounce cooked chicken
   1–2 tablespoons cooked carrots
   ½ teaspoon margarine or butter
   ½ slice bread

Snack
   4 ounces full-fat yogurt such as Stonyfield Farms YoBaby
   2–3 whole grain crackers

Dinner
>8 ounces whole milk
>½ cup cooked noodles with 2 tablespoons meat sauce
>2 tablespoons cooked green beans
>½ teaspoon margarine or butter, if desired
>¼ cup canned pears, drained and chopped

Snack
>4 ounces whole milk
>6 animal crackers

I WANT TO DO IT MYSELF!
BUILDING SELF-FEEDING SKILLS

One- and two-year-olds are thrilled with their newfound physical prowess, including learning how to put things in their mouth. Until they hone this skill at about eighteen months or so, you'll be largely responsible for getting the majority of the meal into your child's mouth. Even so, your child will surely want to join in the feeding process, and should be encouraged to join in, no matter how messy it gets. She may not be able to verbalize it, but a toddler's body language and crying fits will let you know that she wants to feed herself. Self-feeding builds a child's confidence and helps her practice her fine motor skills. As she matures, the connection between her brain and her body movements is enhanced, and her ability to self-feed markedly improves.

In My Experience
It's a Messy Job . . .

Emma loves to feed herself. Her ability to use a spoon and a small fork (but mostly fingers) is liberating for me, unless I am in a rush or feel like keeping her semiclean. Most of the time Emma ends up wearing half of whatever she's eating, especially if it's liquid at room temperature. I know that I should be more patient, but when she's spooning the likes of yogurt and melted ice cream into her mouth and then rubbing whatever got on her hands and face into her hair, I start thinking about cleanup. Here's what I do to avoid getting as frustrated when I'm in a hurry to finish the meal and minimize the mess. I bring two spoons to the table, one for me and one for her. I let her eat, and when there's a lull in the action, I feed her some of her food, which she readily accepts.

CHOKING HAZARDS

Children four and under run the greatest risk for choking. Any food that blocks a child's small airway and cuts off her oxygen supply can lead to death. Some foods are more dangerous than others. Slippery food or foods that are hard, round, and don't dissolve easily in saliva are a kid's worst nightmare.

Aside from avoiding dangerous foods, watching children closely when they eat helps, too. Never leave a youngster unattended when he is eating. Kids can choke when they overstuff their mouths, or when they run around with a mouth full of food. Don't let children eat in the car, either. There may be no way for you to help a youngster dislodge food from his throat during a car ride, especially if you are the only adult present.

Help keep kids out of harm's way by avoiding the following foods. Read the list carefully. Chances are, some hazardous foods will come as a big surprise.

- Nuts
- Seeds
- Popcorn
- Snack chips and puffs
- Pretzels
- Raw carrots
- Raisins and other small dried fruit such as cranberries, blueberries, and cherries
- Whole grapes*
- Fresh or frozen blueberries
- Melon balls
- Marshmallows
- Large chunks of meat, poultry, and hot dogs*
- Peanut butter and other nut butters
- Hard candy and cough drops
- Chewing gum
- Jellybeans
- Gumdrops and other soft jelly candies
- Gummy bears and other hard jelly candies

*Chop grapes and coin-shaped hot dog slices into quarters.

BREAKING AWAY FROM BOTTLES

I always dreamt that my babies would go directly from breastfeeding to drinking out of a cup, with no bottles in between. Well, it never happened that way. Tom and I were left with the task of weaning three children, all of whom loved their bottles and did not give them up readily. Everybody has to do things that he or she is loathe to do as a parent. Mine was taking away my children's baby bottles. Why? It comes down to convenience. It's simpler to track a child's milk consumption with bottle-feeding, and I found it easier to soothe my children before bed with a bottle of warm milk so that they drifted off to guaranteed sleep.

But your child cannot go on forever drinking from baby bottles, for a number of reasons. Relying on a bottle for beverages may interfere with a toddler's ability to drink from a cup. Kids can come to depend on the bottle to feel full. In doing so, they may easily consume too much milk and not enough solid foods, which contain a variety of nutrients. The bottle could become a source of additional calories, too, leading to an overweight child, especially when she's allowed to suck on a bottle at will. Of course, you should never permit a child to sleep with a bottle of milk or juice in his mouth, because it promotes tooth decay.

So, how do you banish the bottle? Gradually, for the most part. Some children give it up themselves (I should be so lucky), while others hold fast. Here's a trick I used with Emma, who had her last bottle at nearly sixteen months of age. I warmed her milk slightly and gave it to her in her sippy cup just before bedtime. I was sure she would resist the change, but I was wrong. She took about an ounce, calmly gave me back the cup, stuck her thumb in her mouth, and went quietly into her crib without a whimper. A few nights of that and she gave up milk before bed in favor of reading books.

SNACKS: WHAT AND HOW MUCH

Remember when you fed your baby every three hours or so? His stomach was tiny, so he needed to refuel frequently to keep up with the nutrient demands of his rapid growth. Your child's stomach capacity has increased some, but it's still limited enough for him to require two or three daily between-meal snacks, provided he's hungry for them.

The best snacks are mini meals, not meal wreckers, so start small and give your child just enough to hold him until the next meal. Of course, this does not always work out perfectly with one- and two-year-olds, since their appetites are erratic. It's OK if your child ends up eating a bigger snack as long as it's healthy. Left to their own devices, kids usually curb food consumption at the next meal. Here are some snack options for toddlers and older children.

- Natural cheese such as cheddar, Havarti, or Swiss

- Fruit juice (limit to 4 ounces a day)

- Milk (full-fat for up to two years old)
- Yogurt (full-fat for up to two years old)
- Hard-cooked eggs
- Cottage cheese (full-fat for up to two years old)
- Tuna
- Whole grain breads and crackers
- Fruit (with the exception of whole grapes)
- Graham crackers
- Plain cookies such as animal crackers
- Pudding (made with full-fat milk)
- Dry cereal or a small bowl of cereal with milk
- Vegetable juices
- Well-cooked vegetables such as a sliced, peeled sweet potato
- Tortillas

LIMITED EATERS: SURVIVAL TIPS FOR PARENTS

Time was, your infant ate with little encouragement from you. Your two-year-old is a different matter, however. You find yourself cajoling, begging, and playing games to interest your son in food. You become locked in a battle of wills, and before you know it, you've branded your child a picky eater for his lack of interest in food.

Not so fast. Calling a child picky because he or she won't eat the foods that you want him to when you want him to isn't entirely fair. *Picky* is a negative term that overlooks what is really going on with a toddler. Let's call such children "limited eaters" instead. Limited eaters don't like a wide array of foods, or they may show a general disinterest in eating for weeks or months on end.

There is a tendency to overreact to a toddler who does not want to eat. Rejecting foods has nothing to do with you or your parenting skills, so don't take it personally. One- and two-year-olds are more often interested in their surroundings than they are in food.

As children age, they learn quickly that refusing food gets a rise out of you that they may actually regard as entertainment. So it behooves parents early on to learn to relax about a child's supposed finicky attitude toward food. Here are some tips for doing just that.

The Do's and Don'ts of Getting Your Child to Eat

- Don't allow grazing. When children have access to food all day long, they may lose interest at mealtime and demand certain highly appealing foods or just refuse the foods they would normally eat if hungry.

- Do serve meals and small snacks at regular intervals to whet a young child's appetite and put off "picky" eating.
- Don't fear nutritional inadequacy. A parent once complained to me about her daughter's limited eating, prompting me to ask just what her child consumed on a regular basis. Turns out, the child's meals and snacks had a lot going for them, even if they lacked an array of foods. Her daughter's diet had no glaring nutrient deficiencies, largely because it contained at least one food from each of the five food groups that she ate in sufficient amounts every day.

    Another thing to consider with kids: While experts, including myself, talk about daily requirements, what's really important is a child's intake over a few days or even a week. That's good news, because a toddler's eating tends to be all over the place. They may fill up on fruit on Monday and Tuesday, then not be interested again until Friday.
- You are the parent, ergo, you are the boss, and you decide what to eat. Does that mean you should serve food your family dislikes in the name of good health? Well, sometimes it works out that way, especially when kids are trying out new foods. They may reject a novel food initially (research shows as many as ten times), then come to love it, and even (dare we hope?) request it. Serving dinners that most family members favor cuts down on the aggravation of food rejection. But if I lived by that rule, we'd be eating chicken cutlets, mashed potatoes, and mandarin oranges every night of the week. You can allow kids to make some food choices without losing control, however. Choosing food for the family is empowering for a child but should not be overdone. Once a week, I allow Hayley and Hannah to decide on dinner, and we usually end up eating pancakes, French toast, or pizza.
- Do capitalize on favorites. Hannah is by far my most limited eater, especially when it comes to vegetables. But she does love potatoes, and she'll tolerate corn. That's why I serve one of those two vegetables with most dinners, alongside a small amount of another less-acceptable vegetable such as broccoli or cauliflower.
- Don't become a short-order cook. Your children won't starve because they don't like tonight's entree. When a kid turns up his nose at what you have to offer, letting him "order" a favorite food for dinner sets a precedent you had better be prepared to live with for a long time. Serve at least one food that everyone likes at each meal, such as bread, rice, potatoes, or pasta; fruit; and milk or cheese, so that you can rest assured your child is getting some nutrition.

- Don't worry that your child is not eating enough. Kids eat when they are hungry. Unlike most adults, young kids have yet to learn to override their instinct to regulate their own eating. For example, babies eat only when they are hungry and stop when they are full. This diminishes with age, when we keep eating because food tastes good rather than because we are hungry. Resist the urge to offer favorite foods to a child who leaves the table without eating his meal. He'll make up for the missing food later.
- Do allow an eating jag to play itself out. Kids typically tire of favorite foods within weeks, so that meal of macaroni and cheese he requests twice a day could be history a month from now. Have faith.
- Do maximize nutrition. When your toddler refuses vegetables, sneak them into the meatloaf or spaghetti sauce she loves, or allow her to dip them into salad dressing. If milk is low on your two-year-old's list of favorite foods, add yogurt to baked goods, top vegetables with melted cheese, or sneak a piece of cheese into her sandwich to boost calcium.

Toddler Turn-Offs

You've made a kid-friendly recipe for dinner and you're sure your two-and-a-half-year-old will love it. But when you present it, she won't even give it a chance. As a rule, toddlers don't particularly like new foods. Toddlers spend their days encountering new things, so they may prefer the comfort of foods they recognize. That's why it's normal for your creations to be rejected on at least one of the following counts.

- Another food is touching it (kids may not want foods to touch)
- Overall appearance
- Color
- Aroma
- Taste
- Texture
- Seasonings

Chapter 7

From Three

to Six Years

Don't they ever get tired?

—Me, *to my husband*

WHAT'S HAPPENING NOW: DEVELOPMENTAL HIGHLIGHTS

Around three, children become increasingly social, more independent, and even more fun to be with than they were before. Preschoolers are particularly playful people who can be quite jovial and entertaining. They love to run, jump, dance, climb, and roughhouse. They find humor in the ridiculous, often laughing easily at the drop of a hat. Clownlike behavior is par for the course.

By three, a child can typically tell you what he wants, even when he can't properly articulate every word or stammers when trying to get through a sentence. With more words at their command, preschoolers can verbalize their feelings. That helps them to work through the tussles they get into with siblings, peers, and parents, and also affords them the ability to voice their food preferences.

A preschooler's increasing physical prowess means more freedom for parents but doesn't decrease the need for supervision. For example, children typically complete toilet training by the end of their third year, which means no more diapers to change. But it does mean you must check to see that junior washes his hands thoroughly after each visit to the bathroom to prevent making himself, and others, ill. One thing's for sure: Your child will have developed self-feeding skills by age three, if not earlier. That means you won't have to spoon-feed him, freeing you up to converse with your youngster and to teach him table manners. Eating with your child with few distractions helps him focus on the task at hand, too.

Four- and five-year-olds are eager, enthusiastic learners with active imaginations. They are curious about numbers and letters and may be capable of reading and writing some simple words by the time they start kindergarten. As your child gets closer to five, you may notice that she is increasingly interested in learning new facts in a spontaneous, fun, and creative way. Now is a good time to get your child interested in food-related activities that not only foster an appreciation of a variety of foods but help her develop simple math and science skills. For example, cooking healthy foods with your child provides practical experience with math, for example, counting out the number of eggs needed, and encourages eye-hand coordination in the measuring of ingredients and in stirring. Setting the table means kids must figure the number of people eating as well as the utensils for each person.

While children ages three through six are relatively agreeable people most of the time, they tend to test their limits. Quite often, mealtime is the battleground. That's why parents must keep their cool, now more than ever.

FEEDING YOUR PRESCHOOLER

As your child moves toward six, his nutrient needs continue to evolve into a more adultlike diet. Pound for pound, youngsters require less energy with increasing age. Since the amount of fat kids need to flourish depends on their calorie intake, fat requirements gradually go down with advancing age, too. In fact, now is a good time to start nudging your child toward a lower fat diet.

Parents often find daily guidelines for fat and calorie intake helpful because they provide a benchmark for a child's progress. While the suggested intakes for calories and fat are based on scientific research, the numbers apply to groups of children, not to individual youngsters. In fact, they are not intended to be used as a guideline for your child. That's because each child's calorie needs are unique. Plus, a preschooler's appetite may be all over the map for a variety of reasons, which makes a daily quota out of the question. It's best to loosely monitor calorie and fat consumption over the course of a few days, or even a week. Don't become too concerned unless a pediatrician diagnoses your preschooler as underweight or overweight, or at high risk for heart disease.

Milk: When, What, and How?

Starting at age two, most children can safely drink reduced-fat milk, including 1% low-fat and 2% reduced-fat. That's because your youngster requires less of the fat and cholesterol concentrated in full-fat milk than she did during her first two years. That's not to say that you must serve skim or 1% low-fat or light milk, however. Your daughter may still need the calories that full-fat dairy products supply. Whatever milk you choose, make sure your child drinks enough to get the calcium required by growing bones. Three-year-olds need 500 milligrams of calcium a day, the equivalent of about 14 ounces of milk or fortified soy beverage. Four-, five-, and six-year-olds need much more: 800 milligrams of calcium daily, or about 24 ounces of milk or fortified soy beverage. (See page 29 for information on calcium-rich foods for kids who don't drink enough milk.)

Fat: Don't Go Too Low

For the first six months of life, breast milk or infant formula provided the primary fat source for your baby. During infancy, your baby needs about 50 percent of his calories from fat in order to get the calories and essential fats to fuel brain and body development. By the time kids reach the age of five, experts say that they require only about a third of their calories as fat, however. That's the same amount as adults should eat for good health.

Yet, in spite of the recommendation for slowly reducing fat in a child's diet until it accounts for about 30 percent of the total calories consumed, parents should know that there are no proven benefits to going lower than the suggested amount. In fact, restricting a preschooler's fat intake can be dangerous. According to the AAP, consuming less than 30 percent fat calories is typically unnecessary, and may make it difficult for children to get the calories and other nutrients they need to grow and develop properly. That's not to say that higher fat diets are always healthier ones. Depending on the fat sources, high-fat diets can be quite unhealthy for kids and can prove just as detrimental to growth as very low-fat eating regimens.

Parents who serve a variety of high- and low-fat foods are on the right track with their children's eating. It makes little sense to exclude nutrient-packed kid favorites such as beef, cheese, and peanut butter based on their fat content. In fact, it's foolish to omit these foods, since they are also rich in vitamins and minerals. Cutting back on snack chips, French fries, and cookies makes more sense for controlling fat because these foods lack nutritional benefit.

Counting on Calories

This may come as a surprise, but depending on their age, preschoolers require as many calories as some sedentary men and women.

A three-year-old needs an average of 1,300 calories daily, or about 45 calories for every pound of body weight. Four- and five-year-olds require on the order of 1,300 to 1,800 calories a day. That translates to about 41 calories per pound of body weight. Although your preschooler may need as many calories to grow as you do to maintain your weight, when you compare calorie needs on a pound-per-pound basis, youngsters require three times as many calories as adults. Why the difference? They're growing and you're not. That's why a preschooler's energy demands are far greater for their size than an adult's, who is physically mature.

In My Experience
Check Body Image Talk at the Door

Children become keenly aware of their bodies at about age four. At the same time, they may hear negative talk about how you, your babysitter, or someone on television feels about their weight or body shape. Young girls are particularly tuned in to "body talk." That's why you must take care to avoid making negative remarks about your build, your spouse's, or anyone else's you encounter. Surely, few women reading this book are completely satisfied with their bodies, so it may prove difficult to contain your displeasure. But try to keep it to yourself. Four- and five-year-olds are intelligent enough to pick up on your dissatisfaction and wonder about the adequacy of their own bodies. They look to their parents to feel good about themselves. Knowing that you feel positively about your shape provides a certain security. If you are unhappy with your weight or shape, speak with a registered dietitian about changing your eating and exercise habits for the better. Or, discuss your feelings with a mental health professional to help improve your body image.

SET THE TABLE, SET THE STAGE FOR FUTURE FOOD CHOICES

Wouldn't it be great if your four-year-old never again turned up her nose at fruits and vegetables? What parent in her right mind wouldn't jump for joy when her five-year-old drinks the recommended three glasses of milk every day, without the whining? You may even want to hug your daughter when she finally decides she likes the homemade chicken pot pie that she has refused to try the first ten times you served it. (Believe me, I've been there.)

If you want these dream scenarios played out at your table, taking the lead will help. Studies show that adults who consume healthy foods have children who eat a more nutritious diet. It's not enough to simply insist your children finish their chicken or polish off their potatoes—you must, too.

The Role of Model

Little ones are like sponges. They soak up what's going on in their immediate surroundings, including your attitude toward food. Even when it appears that they are not paying attention, kids pick up cues about how to act during mealtimes (for example, that you value staying seated, using your napkin instead of your sleeve to wipe your face, and that it's better to converse with other family members than it is to start a food fight); what foods are held in high regard; and what to think about trying new foods. Providing a feeding environment with a minimum of distractions, including no television or loud music, shows children that mealtimes are important parts of the day meant for more than sharing food. For a breast- or bottle-fed infant, calm surroundings provide a pleasant opportunity to bond with Mom or Dad on a one-to-one basis.

Your enthusiasm for healthy foods goes a long way with your kids. When you dig into a new low-fat casserole recipe, finish your vegetables, and choose fruit over cookies for dessert, your children may do the same. Likewise, when you withhold treats such as candy and ice cream and use them as a bribe for finishing dinner, you send the signal that sweets are bargaining tools, which could prove problematic in the long run.

Parents who regularly offer kids new foods expand their child's food universe. Serving up couscous instead of rice or preparing a roll-up instead of a standard sandwich may sound simplistic to you, but it allows kids to imagine all sorts of food possibilities and may even serve as a conversation starter about how children in other parts of the country or the world eat and live. Dining at restaurants on foods not normally eaten at home, such as Middle Eastern, Thai, or Chinese fare, can do the same to broaden a child's horizons. Try new cuisines. Order take-out. That way, the pressure's off and children seem more willing to relax and try new foods.

Mommy See, Mommy Do

When it comes to eating, kids mimic their parents. It seems that moms hold particular sway over their child's food choices. Researchers say that when mothers pick healthy foods such as milk, their children are more likely to follow suit. The *Journal of the American Dietetic Association* reports that youngsters are more apt to drink milk when their mothers do, too. Other studies corroborate the power of Mom's influence on milk drinking, suggesting that children are less likely to consume milk if their mothers don't drink it, even when Mom insists that her kids drink up.

At three, four, or five, each day of a child's life seems filled with discovery, including how others eat. The people your children see on a regular basis—babysitters, relatives, and peers—expand their ideas about food, as does watching television. Contact with adult caregivers, close relatives, and other children with different eating habits at day care, in nursery school, and in kindergarten affect how children view food. Some of this influence may be positive. Witnessing a peer at nursery school or day care eat a certain fruit or vegetable could spark an interest in that food and lead to a request for it. Eating family style in a day care setting can often result in children willingly eating foods they may refuse at home. My kids are much better eaters at my babysitter's house. Eating with their contemporaries cuts down on fussing and fosters acceptance of a wider variety of foods.

While your influence may wane somewhat as your child becomes increasingly autonomous, how you eat at home tends to serve as the strongest influence on your child's eating habits for life.

In My Experience
Variety Is the Key to Good Health

My parents loved to eat a variety of foods and encouraged me to do the same from the time I was very young. I can't say that I ever looked forward to eating the liver and onions they occasionally served, but I am grateful to my mother and father for ignoring my tearful pleas to ban broccoli (and other yucky veggies) from our house. No go. Their policy was firm: You must try a few bites of any food, no matter how you feel about it. Well, I never warmed up to liver, but I have to say that I am a big broccoli fan. I'm not sure if their influence led to my love of broccoli, but you never know.

FENDING OFF FOOD FITS

Now that he can better communicate his eating preferences, your child may hassle you more than ever about eating. Children who regularly refuse food at mealtimes or demand diversions such as television and toys in order to eat are prone to what I have come to call food fits: They use food to gain attention and to manipulate their parents and caregivers. When adults chronically cave in to crying, screaming children, they perpetuate this behavior. Children crave attention of any type. So when you get upset, it's just as fun for them as when you praise them. Watching your reaction to their refusal to eat may actually be a sport for children who regularly throw food fits.

You can't stop a child from fussing about food. But you can control the way you react to her demands for special foods served in certain ways. The good news is that food fits don't have to turn into full-blown food fights.

Parents rule. Who's the boss of your house? You are. Parents decide what foods come into the home, where to dine out, and what type and how much television preschoolers are allowed to watch. Your child will surely put up a stink when he doesn't get the snack food or soda he wants while on a trip to the super-market, or when she's not allowed to watch her favorite TV show during dinner. Yes, your kids will squawk and there will be times when you back down because you are just too tired to tangle with them. That's to be expected. But try to stand firm as often as possible to reduce food fits.

Be flexible. I just said that you are the decision maker, but you don't have to rule with an iron fist, especially when it comes to sweets and other low-quality foods. It's natural for kids to desire salty, fatty, or sugary fare that possesses few redeeming qualities. Occasionally giving in to a request for creme-filled snack cakes will not destroy your efforts to get your child to eat healthfully in the long term. There are no good or bad foods, only good or bad diets. A child's lifelong eating habits are influenced by the way your family eats most of the time, not by occasional splurges on high-fat foods.

Stay cool. Sometimes, you can't tell how kids will react to eating certain foods, so there's no reason to get uptight beforehand. Here's a case in point:

My oldest daughter, Hayley, was five before she ever ate at a fast food restaurant; Hannah was four. I'm sure you're thinking that my profession precludes me from visiting McDonald's and Burger King, but the truth is that I don't really enjoy burgers and French fries, and that's why I don't take my children to fast food joints. (Donuts and other pastries are a different story, however.) So, how did the girls end up eating fast food? A trip to McDonald's came on the heels of a field trip organized by my day care provider. I thought surely the cat was out of the bag then, and that my kids would hound me to no end for chicken nuggets and fries every time we passed a fast food restaurant. I was wrong. They have never once asked for fast food, despite the fact that they loved the McDonald's meal.

Bore them, but only sometimes. Funny thing about stocking your kitchen with a variety of foods: The more choices kids have, the more they tend to eat. This works for and against a healthy diet. Let's say you keep three types of cookies in the cupboards. Your curious preschooler will be tempted to try them all and will probably eat more than you would like as a result (or surely try by pestering you for extra cookies). If graham or animal crackers are the only cookie option, chances are your child will eat enough to satisfy her hunger and be done with them. However, when it comes to pushing produce, variety pays off. How? Having on hand an array of different fruits and vegetables actually increases the likelihood of your child eating more of these nutritious choices.

Give it time. No one consumes an exemplary diet every day, particularly youngsters prone to erratic eating. A mere 2 percent of children ages two through six eat all of the recommended number of servings every day from the five food groups, according to government consumption studies. So don't judge your child's eating on a daily basis. Look at what your child eats over the period of a week or so before deeming his diet inadequate.

Be positive. Four- and five-year-olds may be ready to hear some simple facts about food and nutrition, particularly how it helps them get big and strong. Focus on foods that your child should eat, such as fruits, vegetables, dairy products, meat, poultry, legumes, and whole grains, rather than what foods to avoid because they are "bad for them." My kids are beginning to pick up on certain connections between food and fitness. When Hannah drinks milk, she feels the bone in her thumb and tells us that it's getting stronger. I know that she doesn't quite fathom the reasons why milk makes for stronger bones, but it will sink in some day.

In My Experience
Turn Off Television

The power of television never fails to amaze me. Every time Hayley and Hannah watch even a few minutes of commercial television (and believe me, that's not often), they ask me to buy some wacky snack food that they saw in a flashy, noisy, kid-appealing ten-second ad. What's a parent to do? Curb your kid's TV time. They'll protest at first, but youngsters gradually become accustomed to the limits you set for time spent watching TV, as well as for the type of programs you allow to come into your home.

Aside from encouraging poor eating habits, television is mesmerizing. Kids who get into the habit of eating in front of the television often consume excess calories because they are not focused on their hunger, so they keep on eating. In addition, excessive television viewing stifles a child's creativity and imagination. And watching TV cuts into time for the physical play that burns calories and helps foster lifelong weight control.

Respect their innate ability to regulate. Babies eat only until they are satisfied. Preschoolers are pretty good at self-regulating their intake, too, when left to their own devices. That's why parents who insist that preschoolers clean their plates are inviting trouble. If you belonged to the Clean Plate Club as a kid, you may believe that your child should polish off everything on her plate, regardless of hunger. If it makes you feel better to see a clean plate, offer very small portions to increase the likelihood that no food will go to waste. There is another approach you can take, however. You could respect your child's hunger level and excuse them from eating when they tell you they are full, regardless of what food is left behind.

Kids don't always abide by an adult's schedule. They don't eat by the clock;

they eat when they are hungry. Take the hour or so before dinner. My kids invariably clamor for food, even as I am rushing to prepare a meal for them. But their small stomachs don't work on my timeline. When they're hungry, they want to eat. I give them a small snack to tide them over, and they typically eat a fine dinner after that. When you dismiss a child's hunger because it comes at an inconvenient time, that sends the message that needing food at the wrong time is bad.

PLANNING MEALS FOR YOUR PRESCHOOLER

Now that he's eating more like an adult, it's easier to formulate meals and snacks for your child. First, you need the basic tools of menu planning. See "Pyramid Power" on page 42 for a detailed explanation of what and how much food to serve to children ages two through six.

A Preschooler's Prerogative

If your preschooler had to choose, what would he eat? Macaroni and cheese, pizza, cereal, and chicken. What would he avoid? Green beans, peas, tomatoes, and casseroles. That's according to a report in the *Journal of the American Dietetic Association* that examined the eating habits of seventy-two preschoolers since two months of age, and compared their nutrient intakes to the recommended levels for good health. Since the most common foods in the diets of children in the study between the ages of two and five years included fruit beverages, carbonated soft drinks, and French fries, it's easy to see why the children's diets fell short for several nutrients. The researchers found the youngsters lacked zinc, folate, vitamin E, and vitamin D. Prevent your child from nutrient shortfalls by offering a wide array of the freshest foods early in life. Broadening their palate early on may put off their becoming accustomed to highly processed, salt-, sugar-, and fat-laden foods, and disdainful of healthier fare such as vegetables.

TROUBLESHOOTING A PRESCHOOLER'S EATING

As kids get older, they tend to accept new foods more easily. I've noticed that Hayley, who is nearly six, has become more adventurous in the past year. There are strategies to improve nutrition while you are waiting for your child to be more accepting of a wide range of foods. Here are some of the most common roadblocks to good nutrition, and some simple solutions.

Your Child Won't Eat Vegetables

Most likely texture and/or taste are the main turn-offs for a vegetable hater. Don't expect vegetable avoiders to chow down on strong-tasting choices such as Brussels sprouts and spinach, no matter how you disguise their flavor with butter or cheese. Unless your child is a toddler who needs softer foods, soggy vegetables may not fly with him, so cook vegetables until they're crisp-tender. Include vegetables as part of soups, casseroles, and meatloaf. Offer vegetable juice instead of fruit juice. To make vegetables more interesting, serve them raw with cheese sauce, yogurt dip, or with salad dressing. Pair up peanut butter or hummus with raw or crisp-tender vegetables and count yourself lucky when they eat that combo. (I am so desperate to get more vegetables into my children that I count hummus and peanut butter as part of their daily required vegetable intake. After all, they are made from plant foods.) Don't count French fries or potato puffs as a vegetable, however. Sure, they start out as potatoes, but by the time manufacturers are done with them, they supply far more fat and far fewer nutrients than in their original form.

Your Child Won't Eat Fruit

Kids usually prefer fruit over vegetables, so your problem may be one of limited intake versus all-out rejection of this food group.

She may not sit and eat an entire banana or pear, but perhaps your preschooler will accept fruit on her cereal, as part of a smoothie (see pages 284–286 for recipes), on top of frozen yogurt or ice cream, or baked into cookies and quick breads (she'll never know!). Serve a fruit puree or applesauce instead of syrup for dipping waffles or pancakes. Bake with applesauce or pureed prunes, bananas, or peaches in place of half the fat in recipes for quick breads, including muffins and pancakes, and in cookies. Shredded zucchini and carrots add texture and color to homemade baked goods. Assemble a fruit/cereal/yogurt parfait in a clear plastic glass for breakfast or snack; it's attractive and enticing. Frozen fruit is novel and may encourage intake. Four-year-old Hannah, who is fickle about fruit, likes to nibbles on frozen melon and peaches. I serve Hannah cereals such as Raisin Bran, where the dried fruit is built in. Hayley loves frozen blueberries on her breakfast cereal, and I rely on them when fresh blueberries are out of season. Kids love to dip their foods, so try cubed fruit with yogurt dip to encourage consumption, or make simple fruit kabobs to pique their interest. Juice is a last resort for fruit avoiders, but limit it to 6 ounces a day (4 ounces when your child is eating other fruits and vegetables).

Preschoolers Fall Short on Produce

You know that few kids clamor for apples and bananas and even fewer pester their parents to prepare spinach and broccoli. But the extent of youngsters' produce avoidance is astounding. A report published in the *Journal of the American College of Nutrition* found that out of 168 preschoolers observed over a five-day period, none ate the recommended five servings of fruits and vegetables. The children in the survey ate far more fruits than vegetables, which is encouraging, unless you consider that fruit juice was counted as a fruit serving. Still, kids seem to prefer fruit over vegetables, which offers hope for pumping up kids' consumption of disease-fighting nutrients, particularly antioxidants.

Scientists at the United States Department of Agriculture Research Center on Aging at Tufts University tested the antioxidant power of dozens of fruits and vegetables. Here are the most potent of the lot based on their research. As you can see, most of them are fruits.

- Blackberries
- Blueberries
- Kale
- Oranges
- Plums
- Raisins
- Raspberries
- Red grapes
- Strawberries

Your Child Won't Drink Milk

Milk is among the most calcium-packed foods going. And milk contains vitamin D. Vitamin D helps the body absorb calcium after digestion and fosters its deposition into the skeleton. Despite milk's many benefits, skipping it does not necessarily make for dietary disaster.

Perhaps presentation is the problem. Some kids do not like to drink a plain glass of milk. Hannah drank only chocolate milk for about a year and a half, yet had no trouble accepting milk on top of her breakfast cereal. Disguise milk as chocolate or strawberry; make your child a fruit smoothie with milk (see page 284 for recipe); or prepare hot chocolate, pudding, and condensed soups, such as tomato, with milk instead of water.

Kids who shun milk can make up for lost calcium with other dairy foods such as yogurt, cheese, and cottage cheese. Fruited yogurt supplies about the same amount of calcium as milk, while plain yogurt supplies about a third more. One and a half ounces of hard cheese such as cheddar, Swiss, or Havarti equals eight ounces of milk for calcium, while cottage cheese contains half as much of the mineral unless fortified with added calcium. Calcium can sneak into foods that won't evoke a fuss from kids. Cheese pizza and macaroni and cheese are calcium-packed kid favorites.

Calcium-fortified foods, such as orange juice, soy and rice beverages, and cereal can make up for missing calcium from dairy foods. (To maximize calcium absorption, purchase brands of juice with added calcium citrate malate. Check the ingredient list.) Tofu processed with calcium sulfate helps meet calcium needs, too; a quarter cup provides nearly as much calcium as 4 ounces of milk.

If milk allergy is the reason why your child does not drink milk, then he or she must avoid all dairy products to head off reactions.

Your Child Won't Eat Meat

Children often reject meat and poultry for their texture; tougher cuts of meat may prove too difficult to chew. Sneak lean ground beef or ground 100 percent turkey or chicken meat into spaghetti sauce, tacos, and burritos for greater acceptance. Should you worry about your non-meat eater's nutrition? That depends. Meat packs protein, but so do plenty of other foods. Eggs, milk, cheese, cottage cheese, yogurt, tuna fish, legumes, and nuts make up for missing protein in a meatless diet, but not for the lack of iron and zinc, which are critical to your child's cognitive development and his overall growth. The likes of beef, pork, and chicken are particularly rich in iron and zinc. Fortified breads, cereals, and other grains contain zinc and iron, but your child may need a vitamin/mineral supplement if he completely avoids meat.

Your Child Eats Too Many Sweets and Other Junk Foods

Don't keep the likes of cakes, cookies, donuts, ice cream, or salty snack foods in the house. That doesn't mean you must deprive your little one of treats, however. Offer healthier alternatives such as mini-muffins, graham crackers, animal crackers, fig bars, and gingersnaps. Popcorn, pretzels, and flavored rice cakes topped with peanut butter or hummus are kid-friendly snacks, too. When my children crave something sweet, I make my own trail mix by combining semisweet chocolate chips, raisins or dried cranberries, and nuts (this snack is for children four and older, given the risk for choking in younger kids). If you don't mind whether they have the real thing, purchase just one treat every few weeks or so and dole it out judiciously. But don't use snack chips or cookies as bribes or rewards. Instead, include them as part of meals and snacks, and stay low key about it. When kids get wind that you think certain foods are special, they start blowing their value out of proportion.

Your Child Drinks Too Much Fruit Juice

Serving juice between meals can wreck your child's appetite. Offer water or milk instead when your child claims to be thirsty. Cap your youngster's juice intake at 6 ounces a day, diluting it with water to extend his juice allowance.

FAMILY MATTERS

Family members influence a child's eating and physical activity patterns and attitudes for life. What children do and how they feel about food has implications for nutrition and overall health. Take a moment to assess your own family's eating and physical activity practices. Place a check mark in the column that best describes your practice.

As a parent, family member, or caregiver, do you . . .

	Always	Usually	Sometimes	Never
Eat meals as a family?	☐	☐	☐	☐
Serve meals and snacks on a regular schedule?	☐	☐	☐	☐
Give your youngster freedom to choose the foods he or she eats?	☐	☐	☐	☐
Respect a child's appetite when he or she has had enough?	☐	☐	☐	☐
Involve children in planning and preparing family food?	☐	☐	☐	☐
Make an effort to keep mealtimes pleasant?	☐	☐	☐	☐
Include snacks as part of the day's eating plan?	☐	☐	☐	☐
Attempt to confine eating to the kitchen, dining room, or another designated place?	☐	☐	☐	☐
Set a good role model with your food decisions?	☐	☐	☐	☐
Avoid rewarding or punishing a child with food?	☐	☐	☐	☐
Give kids enough time to eat?	☐	☐	☐	☐
Turn off the TV while you eat together?	☐	☐	☐	☐

	Always	Usually	Sometimes	Never
Offer foods that appeal to children?	☐	☐	☐	☐
Serve a variety of foods for meals and snacks?	☐	☐	☐	☐
Offer new foods and new combinations?	☐	☐	☐	☐
Avoid forcing a child to eat?	☐	☐	☐	☐
Set a good role model by being physically active?	☐	☐	☐	☐
Limit TV time to one to two hours daily?	☐	☐	☐	☐
Encourage children to play actively?	☐	☐	☐	☐
Enjoy physical activity regularly as a family?	☐	☐	☐	☐

To score, count the number of check marks in each column. Then multiply the number of each answer by these scores:

Each "always" gets 3 points.
Each "usually" gets 2 points.
Each "sometimes" gets 1 point.
Each "never" gets 0 points.

What does your score suggest? If you scored **40 to 60** points, you apply what you know about nurturing positive eating and physical activity patterns.

A score of **20 to 39** suggests you're on the right track for feeding kids and exercising with them, but there's still room to make positive changes in your family's lifestyle.

If you scored less than **20**, you'd be wise to make significant changes in your family's approach to food and physical activity.

Note: ©American Dietetic Association. *"ADA's Complete Food and Nutrition Guide."* Used with permission.

Chapter 8

Getting to Know Food

What's that hanging
from those trees?

—*Hayley, on her first trip to pick apples*

T he objects on the trees were apples, but how would Hayley have known? Until her first outing to a local farm, she thought apples came in a bag from the supermarket.

Few of us grew up on a farm, but it seems like we know more about where food comes from than our children do, or will in the future. In this grab-and-go world, highly processed convenience foods are the norm for kids, who often don't have a clue about the origins of what they are eating.

Why should it matter that children know about food? Interested, informed children are more likely to learn to make a lifetime of wiser food choices, especially during adolescence when access to junk food is greater. And adults who eat better are healthier in the long run.

It doesn't take much to get preschoolers fired up about food. Here are some activities to spark their interest.

Grow it. Seeing a plant go from seedling to something edible provides a sense of accomplishment for kids. A garden, window box, or sunny spot in the house provides the opportunity to teach children about plants as food. Children enjoy choosing what to grow, planting the seeds, watching the plant's progress, and then eating the vegetables several weeks or months later. Older youngsters can be responsible for watering plants and can help Mom and Dad transfer them outside to a sunny spot in your yard or deck.

Hayley and Hannah like to monitor the progress of the plants in our small garden. Cherry tomato plants are a particular favorite. As the tomatoes grow, I point out how they go from green to red as they ripen. My children are not vegetable lovers, but they'll eat homegrown cherry tomatoes. Even though the tomatoes are sweet and juicy, I'm not sure taste is totally responsible for Hannah and Hayley's attraction. Accessibility has a lot to do with it. The girls are about the same size as the tomato plants, and they can reach right in and pick as many as they like. They love it when I ask them to gather tomatoes for our lunch or dinner. Even when they don't eat the tomatoes they have picked for the family, it doesn't matter. The act of caring for the plants and reaping the fruits of their labor helps nurture an appreciation for the fact that food can come from the ground.

Borrow it. When you don't have the space or the time for tending plants, perhaps you can "borrow" the benefits of a garden. For example, the kids love to pick raspberries in my mother's backyard. Only about half of the berries actually make it into the house—they eat the rest. The girls are nowhere near as interested in store-bought raspberries, however.

One of my mother's neighbors plants an enormous garden every year. Aside from raiding it several times a summer (with his permission, of course!), I often take my kids into his yard to check on the progress of the many different types of vegetables he plants there. I'm especially lucky that Bill allows my kids and me to plunder his blueberry bushes, since they are my all-time favorite fruit.

Bringing children to a farm to pick their own apples, pears, berries, or pumpkin is a great family activity. It gets everyone out of doors for fresh air and sunshine and physical activity. Since it's less likely that you will grow fruit than vegetables, picking your own is the way to go for showing kids where fruit originates.

Shop for it. You may not be able to garden or make it to a farm. No matter. Trips to the grocery store teach kids about food, too. Getting your children involved in your weekly shopping can go a long way toward interesting them in healthy eating.

Before you leave the house, take inventory and make a list. Kids love to help with these tasks. I tell Hayley what I need; she asks me how to spell it and then writes it down. I've done a week's worth of shopping based on her lists. Kids can also help you check the cupboards for what you need in the way of healthy staples such as bread, cereal, legumes, pasta, and canned tuna fish. Older children can help you clip coupons, too.

It's best to shop early in the day with children to avoid the crowds. Chances are, you'll be moving slowly as you stroll the aisles. I usually take the kids at 8 A.M. on a Saturday or Sunday morning. I never shop with them around lunch- or dinnertime because it's too crowded in the store and they are usually too hungry or too tired to behave.

Once in the store, get a small shopping cart for your youngster to push, and have him fetch some items as you stroll the aisles together. Pointing out new foods will pique his interest: Let him feel the fuzzy outside of a kiwi, and talk to him about where kiwis come from. That could lead to a request to buy one and try it at home.

It's all well and good when kids clamor for fruits, vegetables, and whole grain cereals while in the supermarket. Kids will invariably request foods that are packed with sugar, salt, and fat, and you'll probably give in to their demands at times. That's OK, but don't let it happen too often. It can become a pattern that's hard to break. And never bribe them with food so that they will behave while you are shopping.

> ## Smart Shopping with Kids
>
> - Begin shopping with children at a very early age to help them get comfortable with the routine.
> - Don't shop on an empty stomach. Go after a meal or a snack to reduce the chances of kids requesting food out of hunger.
> - Make a list and stick to it. When kids clamor for junk foods, tell them those items are not on the list.
> - Don't rush. Shop when you have time to spend talking with your kids about food.
> - Shop once a week. Bringing kids into the supermarket more often only increases their requests for items that are costly and devoid of nutrition.
> - Skip the candy aisle, and head for the candy-free checkout aisles, too.
> - Let kids help unload bags when you get home and put foods into the cabinets they can reach and into the refrigerator. Hayley, Hannah, and Emma love to drag the bags into the kitchen and put away the food. It doesn't always end up in the right places, but that doesn't bother me.

KIDS IN THE KITCHEN

It happens most every night, and sometimes at lunch, too. My back is turned, but the sound is familiar enough. It's Hannah, dragging a chair twice her size up to the kitchen counter. Invariably, the next thing out of her mouth is: "Mommy, can I help?"

Preschoolers love simple and manageable cooking tasks. At the tender age of four, Hannah has been helping me prepare food for the family for well over a year, and making pancakes and waffles with her father on weekends. Cooking together is a way to spend one-on-one time with a child. It's also a learning experience where kids practice counting, hone fine motor skills, and get a shot of self-esteem for their accomplishments. When a child can say he made it himself, it may even serve to increase his interest in a variety of foods.

Kids can, and should, help in the kitchen. After all, the preparation that goes into meals is a family chore that is typically left to Mom. Getting kids to help means less work for you in the long run!

The following is a guide to what each age can do as far as food preparation goes. Since every child's skills are different, make sure to tailor their designated tasks to fit their abilities.

All Ages
- Wash hands in warm, soapy water and dry thoroughly.
- Don't let them touch or eat raw animal foods, including meat, poultry, and seafood; ditto for cookie, cake, brownie, or quick bread batter containing raw eggs. Thoroughly wash with warm water and soap the surfaces and utensils touched by raw animal foods.

Two-and-a-Half- and Three-Year-Olds
- Wash fruits and vegetables
- Peel bananas
- Stir batters
- Cut out cookies from rolled-out dough, with assistance
- Slice with a sturdy plastic knife soft foods such as bananas, mushrooms, cooked and cooled potatoes and sweet potatoes
- Help pour water, sugar, salt, oil, or other ingredients into batter
- Help measure ingredients such as raisins, chocolate chips, and chopped nuts, rice, and other grains

Four- and Five-Year-Olds
- Do everything listed above
- Grease pans
- Get mixing bowls, wooden spoons, and canned ingredients and bring them to the kitchen work space
- Open packages
- Roll out or shape dough for cookies
- Shape dough for pizza
- Fill muffin tins with batter
- Use scissors to trim the ends from green beans or to snip fresh herbs
- Help set the table

"I Made It Myself!"

With some assistance and the right ingredients, kids can concoct delicious and nutritious fare. Here's how.

Juice pops: Help children pour 100 percent fruit juice into plastic ice-pop molds. Cover and freeze.

Fruit yogurt crunch: Children measure out a teaspoon of their favorite jam or jelly and mix with 4 ounces plain yogurt and some crunchy breakfast cereal.

Potato chips: Wash and cut a small white or sweet potato into thin slices and place in a bowl. Children measure a teaspoon of vegetable oil, pour it over the potatoes, and stir to coat. Kids put the potato chips in a single layer on a baking sheet. Parents place the cookie sheet in a 400°F oven for ten minutes; remove when potatoes are tender. Let them sufficiently cool before serving to children.

Snack chips: Older children can use scissors to cut pita bread or tortillas into wedges. Parents place wedges in a toaster oven. Kids can press the "toast" button. Toast lightly and let cool sufficiently. Use for dipping in hummus, peanut butter, or yogurt-based dips.

Ice cream sandwiches: Kids pile 2 tablespoons of slightly softened frozen yogurt or ice cream onto a honey or chocolate graham cracker square, and top with another square. Place in freezer to harden, and enjoy.

Tartar sauce: Have kids measure out a cup of mayonnaise and place into a medium bowl, then add an equal amount of relish, and stir. Serve with fish sticks.

Bean burrito: Children spoon refried beans onto flat tortillas, top with chopped tomato or salsa and grated cheese, roll up, and place in small baking pan. Adults place the pan in a 350°F oven for five to ten minutes, and cool sufficiently.

Personal pizza: Kids top a prepared personal size pizza crust or small tortilla with tomato sauce, grated cheese, and chopped vegetables, then place it on a baking sheet. An adult puts the baking sheet in a 400°F oven for about ten minutes, or until the cheese is melted. Cool, then enjoy.

HEALTHY READING FOR KIDS

Reading to your child promotes her language skills. Plus, kids love hearing the sound of your voice and spending special time with you when reading is the activity. Any of the following books are appropriate for babyhood and beyond.

The Berenstain Bears and Too Much Junk Food by Stan and Jan Berenstain (Random House, 1985)
Blueberries for Sal by Robert McCloskey (Viking Press, 1948)
Bread and Jam for Frances by Russell Hoban (Scholastic Books, 1964)
Eating the Alphabet: Fruits and Vegetables from A to Z by Lois Ehlert (Harcourt Brace Jovanovich, 1989)
Family Dinner by Jane Culter (Farrar, Straus, Giroux, 1991)
Joseph and Nellie, by Bijou Le Tord (Bradbury Press, 1986)
A Kid's Book About Healthy Bones by the Medical Information Group (Medical Information Group, 1997)
The Milkmakers by Gail Gibbons (Macmillan Inc., 1985)
The Very Hungry Caterpillar by Eric Carle (Philomel Books, 1983)

Chapter 9

Feeding Frenzy!
The How-To's of
Healthy Family Fare

To avoid conflict, sometimes parents go for the easiest route, like feeding kids what they want rather than what they need. I know I've done it.

—Janice, mother of two

Thisis may be your first baby, or your fourth. Whatever the case, the frantic pace of day-to-day family life makes feeding one or more children a daunting task.

What with juggling work and family, eating right often gets lost in the shuffle. Lack of time is an enormous barrier to good nutrition that seems to get worse as your family grows and the children mature. Perhaps you made your own baby food when your first child came along, but now that there are three kids who need your care, you simply don't have the time. Long days at work for you and your spouse may mean your family's evening meal often consists of takeout fare that's high in calories, fat, and sodium but lacking in the vitamins, minerals, and fiber children and adults require.

You've got a lot on your plate. Even if you do have the feeding thing down pat—that is to say, you have the time to shop and prepare perfectly well-balanced meals and snacks for your family—your kids may not cooperate with all of your good intentions. Children seem to change their eating routines as often as they change their clothes. Growth spurts and fussiness top the list. Despite the challenges, your most important job as a parent is serving the healthiest fare possible. Good nutrition affects your child's learning ability and physical growth. This chapter provides a meal-by-meal plan that helps busy parents put nutritious foods on the table fast.

BREAKFAST BENEFITS

Breakfast has been called the most important meal of the day, and with good reason. While every meal counts toward good nutrition, the facts are on the table: Eating in the morning has positive effects on health and on kids' ability to learn.

What's a nutritious breakfast? A meal consisting of foods from at least two of the five food groups is healthiest, but the truth is that noshing on nearly any food in the morning is better than none, especially when it come to kids.

It's a good idea to get your child into the habit of eating breakfast before he begins kindergarten. That's because youngsters who eat breakfast tend to fare better in school and have a healthier overall diet. Hunger makes it harder to keep your mind focused on learning, no matter what your age. In fact, studies show breakfast skippers are often more irritable and have shorter attention spans. Here's a possible explanation. When you forgo eating in the morning, blood glucose levels drop. Glucose is the fuel cells need to function, so brain cells become particularly sluggish when glucose concentrations are insufficient. Without adequate energy, young minds get fuzzy, hampering concentration and memory.

Without the morning meal, kids are hard-pressed to meet daily nutrient needs, too. A simple, easy-to-fix meal of fortified cereal with eight ounces of milk and six ounces of orange juice provides substantial amounts of a variety of nutrients, particularly B vitamins, vitamins C and D, calcium, folic acid, and iron if the cereal is fortified with it.

Navigate the Morning Rush

With all the promise of the morning meal, why don't more kids eat breakfast? You're probably pressed for time in the morning, and so are your children. Simplify your morning routine with these tips:

- Get up ten minutes earlier.
- Give up morning television and computer games in favor of concentrating on the task at hand: eating breakfast.
- Stock the kitchen with healthy, quick-to-fix breakfast foods, including cereal, waffles, pancakes, milk, juice, cottage cheese, bread, fruit, and peanut butter.
- The night before kindergarten or nursery school, help kids pack their school bags and decide what to wear the next day to reduce the morning chaos.

On the Menu: Not Your Basic Breakfast Foods

Your kids may balk at traditional breakfast foods, but that doesn't mean they must go without. Here's how to jazz up the morning meal.

- Split a bagel. Spread each half with peanut butter and sprinkle with raisins. Serve with milk.
- Warm up leftover pizza or serve it cold. Have kids sip juice to go with it.
- Combine a soft pretzel, string cheese, and fresh fruit for breakfast.
- Serve 8 ounces of yogurt, a piece of toast, and juice.
- Mix it up with a hard-boiled egg, small roll, and a piece of fruit.

- Heat a freshly made or frozen pancake, spread with peanut butter, top with sliced banana, and roll up.
- Layer one or two slices of turkey breast and one slice cheese on a tortilla or colorful sandwich wrap. Roll up. Serve with juice or with fruit.
- Concoct a breakfast parfait with layers of fruit yogurt; sliced fresh fruit; and crunchy, iron-fortified cereal. Kids love this in an ice cream cone.
- Swirl applesauce and raisins into warm oatmeal. Serve with milk.
- Combine in a blender until frothy: ½ cup lemon yogurt, ½ cup milk, dash vanilla extract, and 2 ice cubes. Complement with a slice of whole grain toast.
- Scramble an egg, stuff into half a pita pocket, and top with ketchup or mild salsa, if desired. Serve with juice or fruit.
- Puree chunks of peaches, pears, or apples in the blender or food processor. Thin with fruit juice to desired consistency. Use instead of syrup on fat waffles and pancakes. Add milk to make a meal.
- Mix cottage cheese with chopped peaches, pears, or apples. Spread on whole wheat crackers or toast.

LIVELY LUNCH

In our household, lunch is fairly straightforward. It's one of the easiest meals for me to prepare. Hannah and Hayley would eat the same sandwich every day for months on end without tiring of it. For example, we just finished a stretch of peanut butter and marshmallow creme sandwiches, fruit, and milk. Much to my pleasure and surprise, they have recently begun branching out into tuna fish and grilled cheese.

An ideal lunch consists of adequate servings from at least three food groups. A sandwich, fruit or vegetable, and milk is so appealing because it includes foods from four of the five possible food groups. I'm not a stickler for traditional "lunch" foods, however. Some children don't like sandwiches. No problem. As long as youngsters eat a balanced meal and a varied diet, that's fine by me. Try these alternatives to the standard lunch fare:

- Whole wheat crackers, string cheese, applesauce, milk
- Whole grain roll with butter or margarine, hard-boiled egg, carrot sticks (give chopped, cooked carrots to kids under the age of four to prevent choking), milk
- Yogurt, crackers, and cantaloupe
- Cottage cheese, whole grain roll with butter or margarine, cherry tomatoes (cut up for kids under four)
- Veggie burger, whole grain roll, fruit, milk

Stuck in a Sandwich Rut?

When kids are stuck on the same old sandwich, try to vary one aspect instead of altering it completely all at once.

- Try whole grain breads including pita, tortillas, and colorful sandwich wraps as a change of pace.
- Vary sandwich fillings: offer a veggie burger, turkey, tuna fish, chicken, or beef. Tantalize taste buds by adding chopped celery or water chestnuts to tuna salad or combining diced chicken with grapes when making chicken salad. Sliced bananas and apples or shredded carrots make colorful additions to sandwiches.
- Condiments such as mustard may be too strong tasting for kids, but mayonnaise, salad dressings, and cranberry sauce can be used to dress up sandwiches.

DINNERTIME DILEMMA

I dread dinnertime. Without question, dinner is the most difficult meal of the day for me. It's when I juggle the nutritional needs and eating preferences of three children while trying to prepare an interesting, healthy meal for Tom and myself. Throughout the day, the dietitian in me has kept mental tabs on what each child has eaten and what remains to be consumed at dinner. Thoughts like "Hannah drank juice at lunch and should drink milk with dinner"; "Hayley hasn't had fruit all day"; and "Emma needs more protein" fly through my head as I struggle to get dinner on the table in a timely fashion.

Until recently, dinnertime found me preparing three different meals, despite the fact that I am no short-order cook. So why did I spend so much of my time in the kitchen? Emma was an infant, so she didn't eat too much table food without a lot of assistance. And Hannah and Hayley prefer plainer foods than Tom and I like to eat, so there was no way that a combination dish of garlic-laden chicken, broccoli, and ziti would fly with them.

Although I'm against catering to each family member's food preferences, I do have my limits. I prefer to serve meals that nearly everyone likes. There are three dinners the whole family will eat without any fuss, but that doesn't mean that I will serve French toast, pancakes, and macaroni and cheese night after night.

Eating jags keep me on my toes, too. The girls may all favor certain foods, but hardly ever on the same day, especially when it comes to fruits and vegetables. Hannah and Hayley like mashed potatoes, but Emma won't touch them (even though she's been exposed to them more than the recommended ten times already); Hayley eats asparagus, but Hannah hates it; Hannah prefers her pears peeled and sliced, while Hayley will eat whole pears, and so on. Thank goodness Tom likes nearly everything I make for dinner!

Supper, Simplified

By the end of the day, you're tired and little ones are cranky. You want to put a well-balanced meal on the table, but you can't always spare the time, nor do you have the energy it takes to prepare dinner. That's why you so often settle for the same meal, or for high-fat, low-nutrient convenience fare. Good news: Dinner doesn't have to be elaborate to be nutritious and satisfying. (Mine never is.) These suggestions can simplify the daily process of getting a good meal on the table.

Consult the Family Calendar

The whereabouts of family members can determine what's for dinner. Even at this tender young age, your kids may have activities that cut into dinnertime, or your spouse or partner may be working late or out of town during the week. When Tom or I won't be home for dinner, the family eats much more simply. That's when we order in pizza and have it with milk and fruit, or cook up scrambled eggs or a cheese omelet to go along with toast and vegetables.

Shop Regularly

It's 6:00 P.M., and there's not a fruit or vegetable in your refrigerator. You can't prepare the quick and healthy dinners that you dream of when your kitchen is not stocked with the fixings.

After perusing the family calendar, devise a weekly dinner menu to avoid ordering takeout when time gets tight and you're too tired to cook. While you're at it, purchase some breakfast and lunch items to take to the office. For the inconvenience of preparing your own breakfast and lunch, you'll save a lot of money: A week's worth of takeout coffee and bagel with cream cheese and commercially prepared salads or sandwiches for lunch can easily cost upwards of $120 a month per person, depending on where you live.

Keep your cupboards crammed with ingredients for nutritious meals by posting a running list on a bulletin board or refrigerator. Write down items you need as they are used up. Take some time on the weekend to make out a shopping list or use the one on page 151 (see "Do You Have What It Takes?") as a template. Once you're in the supermarket, don't deviate from your list unless it's to purchase an item you need but forgot to write down, or you find a sale item you cannot pass up. Unit pricing can help you get the most for your money. When comparing products such as poultry and salad dressing, check the price per unit, which is typically in pounds or ounces. Unit prices are often posted on the package (as in the case of fresh meat and seafood) or on shelves directly under the food.

Think Ahead

Prepare at least one meal on the weekend to serve as the basis for other meals throughout the coming weeks; store extra food in airtight containers for future use. Roast a chicken or a small turkey breast or prepare a double batch of stew, soup, or lasagna to get a jump on weeknight dinners. Add a grain and vegetable to leftover poultry for a fast meal; make chicken or turkey salad sandwiches or fajitas and serve with salad or soup; and take the chicken or turkey carcass and prepare soup from it. Soups and stews serve as the centerpiece at dinnertime with crusty bread and a salad as partners (use prewashed salad mixes for faster preparation). When cooking dinner on a weekday, *always* make enough for another meal. Whipping up double batches saves time. It does wonders to know that you have a delicious meal for the following night, too.

Eat Breakfast for Dinner

Pancakes and waffles are two foods our entire family loves, even at dinnertime. There is nothing wrong with eating the likes of omelets, scrambled eggs, or breakfast cereal for supper. In fact, traditional breakfast foods provide the basis for a fast and healthy meal, especially when kids are hungry and you're too pooped to cook. Don't forget to add fruit or vegetables, milk, and a grain, when necessary. For example, serve up French toast with fruit and milk; scrambled eggs with toast and a fruit or vegetable and milk; or blueberry pancakes and milk.

Capitalize on Convenience

They cost more, but prepared foods save time. Depending on what they are, store-bought foods can serve as the centerpiece of a meal, or as a side dish. Pair up a roasted chicken with fresh or frozen vegetables and a quick-cooking grain such as packaged couscous. You can use takeout pizza as the beginnings of a healthy meal, too. Order a thin crust cheese pie and combine it with a large hearty salad made from packaged salad greens, grated carrots, and cherry tomatoes. Baby carrots can be microwaved for a quick and healthy side dish. You can skip the peeling and chopping when you rely on prepared butternut squash or potatoes your grocer sells in the produce aisle.

Do You Have What It Takes?

Parents are pressed for time. That's why you don't typically make meal plans and shopping lists and sometimes come up short for healthy ingredients. Use this list as a first step toward keeping on hand the ingredients you need to fix delicious and nutritious fare. Make a copy every week and add and delete items to fit your family's needs.

Breads and Grains
- Whole grain bread
- Fortified infant cereal
- Fortified pasta
- Fortified rice
- Fortified whole grain cereal with at least 3 grams fiber per serving
- Prepared pizza crust
- Frozen whole grain waffles or pancakes
- Tortillas
- Sandwich wraps
- Pretzels
- Pancake mix
- Cornbread muffin mix
- Other grains

Fruits and Vegetables
- Apples
- Bananas
- Berries
- Broccoli
- Carrots
- Cauliflower
- Corn
- Eggplant
- Frozen fruits and vegetables such as blueberries, corn, peas, and frozen stir-fry vegetable mixes
- Grapes
- Kiwi
- Lettuce
- Melon
- Onions
- Pears
- Potatoes
- Romaine lettuce
- Spinach
- Squash
- Sweet potatoes
- Tomatoes
- Zucchini
- Jars of pureed fruits and vegetables for baby
- Other fruits and vegetables

Milk Products
- Milk
- Cheese
- Cottage cheese
- Evaporated milk
- Powdered milk
- Yogurt
- Other dairy products

(continued)

Meat and Other High-Protein Foods
- Canned, dried, or frozen legumes
- Tofu
- Fortified soy beverage
- Canned tuna fish
- Peanut butter and other nut butters
- Whole roasting chicken or turkey (save carcass to make soup)
- Eggs
- Skinless chicken or turkey breast
- 100 percent ground chicken or turkey meat
- Lean cuts of beef and pork
- Other protein foods

Condiments
- Balsamic or red wine vinegar
- Butter or margarine
- Canola oil
- Jelly or jam
- Ketchup
- Low-sodium chicken bouillon cubes or packets
- Mayonnaise
- Mustard
- Olive oil
- Relish
- Salad dressing
- Soy sauce
- Other condiments

WHY EAT TOGETHER?

Family meals are much more than a time for kids to sit at the same table with siblings and parents. Kids crave ritual and family meals are a part of a routine they can count on and take comfort in. Mealtimes may be one of the only parts of the day when children get to talk with their parents without a lot of other distractions, including the television and radio. In fact, research shows dinner conversation boosts a child's vocabulary, which could translate into improved academic performance down the line. Lingering at the table to talk allows you to catch up on what's happening with your kids. Go around the table and encourage each child to tell the rest of the family about her day, and don't leave out baby. Infants love to hear your voice and to make eye contact with you. Talking to them about anything strengthens their language development.

Breaking bread with your children allows them to model your behavior, which is necessary for instilling good manners. Eating together offers children the chance to see their parents eat a variety of foods, too.

It's not always possible for all family members to be together at every meal.

Don't worry about not being there all the time. Experts say that while eating family meals together fosters closeness and development, time spent together is what really matters. Studies done at the University of Minnesota and the University of North Carolina found parents' presence in the home was associated with reduced drug use, sex, violence, and emotional distress in teenagers.

Although your children are a long way from adolescence, now is the time to get into the habit of spending time together without distraction. If you cannot be present for mealtime, encourage your child to sit with you while you eat when you return home. Up until your child goes to elementary school, his life is relatively free of extracurricular activities. It will only get harder to gather everyone around the table for dinner as time goes on. So take advantage of this time of your child's life and try to have as many meals together as possible.

FOOD LABEL LINGO

Changes in the laws governing the nutrition facts and figures on food labels and health claims concerning food make the information on food packages consistent and more well defined than ever. The Nutrition Facts Panel takes on a modified form when it appears on foods intended for young children. Here's how the labels differ:

- Infant food labels do not list calories from fat, saturated fat, or cholesterol content. This is done to avoid focusing on these nutrients as ones to control in a child's diet. During the first two years of life, babies require fat and cholesterol to fuel their growth and for brain development. There is hardly ever a medical reason for limiting these nutrients.
- Serving sizes are based on average amounts that children eat at any given time.
- The Daily Value (DV) provides information about how a serving of that food fits into a reference diet. The Nutrition Facts Panel on foods intended for children excludes % DV for fat, cholesterol, sodium, potassium, carbohydrate, and fiber because there are no established DV for these nutrients in children under the age of four.
- Manufacturers are not allowed to make health claims about the benefits of foods intended for young children.

Labeling Speak

This term . . .	Means that . . .
Calorie Free	The product contains fewer than 5 calories per serving.
Low Calorie	Each serving supplies 40 or fewer calories.
Light or Lite	The food contains a third fewer calories or 50 percent less fat. If the food derives more than half its calories from fat, then its fat level must by reduced by 50 percent or more to make this claim.
Light in Sodium	It has half the sodium of its counterparts.
Fat Free	The product contains a half-gram of fat per serving, or even less.
Low Fat	You won't get any more than 3 grams of fat per suggested portion.
Low Saturated Fat	One gram or less per portion is saturated fat.
Cholesterol Free	This product serves up 20 milligrams or less cholesterol and 2 grams saturated fat, or less.
Sodium Free	A serving provides fewer than 5 milligrams of sodium.
Very Low Sodium	A portion contains 35 milligrams or less of sodium.
High Fiber	A portion of this food serves up at least 5 grams of dietary fiber.
Sugar Free	Less than half a gram of sugar per serving.
High, Rich In, or Excellent Source Of	One serving supplies at least 20 percent of the DV for a certain nutrient.
Good Source	A portion provides at least 10 percent of the DV for a certain nutrient.

What's It All About?

Food labels are full of useful information. Here's how to get more out of them.

- **% DV.** These figures provide a basis for determining how a serving of a certain food fits into your daily requirements for selected nutrients, and, ultimately, whether it's worth eating. For instance, an 8-ounce glass of milk supplies 30 percent of the DV for calcium, which happens to be 1,000 milligrams. That means eight ounces of milk provides 300 milligrams of calcium, a considerable bang for the buck. The % DV is the best estimate of how a serving of processed food helps satisfy daily nutrient needs.
- **Health claims.** A health claim makes reference to the potential benefits of that particular food, or of a nutrient found in it. Example: Eating high-fiber grain products may help prevent some cancers. Health claims are typically positioned on the front of food packages.

Look for These Terms on Packaged Meat, Poultry, and Seafood

This term . . .	Means that . . .
Lean	In a 3-ounce portion, there are less than 10 grams of total fat, fewer than 4.5 grams saturated fat, and no more than 95 milligrams cholesterol.
Extra Lean	This food contains less than 5 grams of total fat and fewer than 2 grams of saturated fat, and no more than 95 milligrams cholesterol per three ounces.

Chapter 10

Super Foods
for Kids
(and Adults)

All foods fit into
a balanced diet.

—*The Dietitian's Mantra*

All foods may fit. But let's be frank. Some foods are better than others, especially for children.

When you are trying to feed a growing family on a tight budget and limited time, eating foods that offer the biggest bang for the buck takes precedence. That's why choosing the cheapest, easiest-to-prepare foods packed with the most nutrition is the way to go. To that end, I have put together my list of favorite, tasty super foods for children that won't break the bank.

It's difficult to come up with a short list of top foods because so many qualify as great choices for growing bodies. So how did I decide? First and foremost, foods had to be kid-friendly *and* filled with nutrients to make the grade. That rules out the likes of kale, Brussels sprouts, and liver, for example. They may pack nutrients, but nearly all youngsters turn up their noses at the prospect of eating them. Once a food made it past the primary criteria of great taste and good nutrition (according to my taste buds), I looked at how it fit in with the other entries. I needed to narrow down the list while concentrating on providing a variety of selections for parents and children, which is why there is an array of choices. You'll see foods from every food group listed here.

What about the foods left off the list? I couldn't include everything, just the choices I thought most worthy. So if your family favorites are missing, that doesn't necessarily make them bad-for-you foods. Admittedly, the list lacks dozens of nutritious foods, most notably fruits and vegetables. Yet, all plant foods have something wonderful to offer kids by way of nutrition, so you should never rule out any of them.

Just because they're good for you doesn't mean children will eat all of the super foods highlighted here. Chances are, your kids will reject many of my favorites on the grounds of taste, but keep trying. Some day your little tike will surprise you when he actually asks to snack on sweet potatoes or demands hummus for lunch. Hey, stranger things have happened. See the recipe section for ways to use many of these super foods.

SWEET POTATOES

Why they're good for a growing body: These sweet tubers taste great warm or cold, and they're pretty to look at, too. A sweet potato provides carbohydrate, potassium, vitamin C, folate, fiber, and carotenoids, substances that the body uses to make vitamin A and to fight off disease.

How to serve: Slice cold, cooked, peeled sweet potatoes for a snack or side dish. Mash cooked sweet potatoes with orange juice for an extra boost of vitamin C and folate. Thinly slice peeled sweet potatoes, toss in canola oil, and bake. Serve warm or cold as a potato chip substitute. Cut peeled sweet potatoes into wedges and roast along with sliced apples or white potatoes. Bake a crustless sweet potato pie and serve with low-fat vanilla frozen yogurt for a calcium-rich treat.

When to begin offering: There's no reason why sweet potatoes can't be one of the first vegetables your child eats during infancy. My kids loved pureed sweet potatoes straight out of the jar. You can make your own by thoroughly mashing or pureeing a cooked skinless tuber with breast milk or infant formula. Make sure the consistency is right for your infant's developmental stage.

BROCCOLI

Why it's good for a growing body: Broccoli is packed with energy-producing carbohydrate, as well as fiber, a carbohydrate with no calories, but lots of health benefits. Broccoli also supplies numerous vitamins and minerals in healthy doses, including calcium, potassium, folate, and carotenoids that foster peak eyesight, ward off cell damage, and serve as the raw material for vitamin A production in the body.

How to serve: Kids are funny about broccoli. Hannah and Hayley liked it when they were just out of infancy, but it fell out of favor with both of them when they reached two or three. Broccoli's strong taste can be off-putting, which is why I let my children slather it with reduced-fat salad dressing. Broccoli is so beneficial that I will let them eat it however they want. Your children may take to broccoli more easily than mine did (and then, didn't), in which case serving it raw or lightly steamed is your best bet. In fact, cooking broccoli until it's just crisp-tender frees up some of the beneficial phytochemicals, helping the body to better absorb them. When children refuse plain broccoli, try making soup out of it (see recipe, page 278).

When to begin offering: Babies can try pureed broccoli at six months or so.

WHOLE GRAINS

Why they're good for a growing body: Whole grains are rich in fiber and vitamin E, usually very low in fat, and nearly always devoid of cholesterol (as are most grain products). The germ and outer coating in wheat and other grains harbors many of its valuable nutrients. That's why breads, cereals, and other products produced from whole grains retain the bulk of their nutritive value, as opposed to refined grain foods such as white bread and certain breakfast cereals. Whole grains are typically fortified with folic acid, B vitamins, iron, and zinc, which only adds to their appeal. Some whole grain breakfast cereals contain added calcium and vitamin D, too. Studies show that whole grains provide protection against certain chronic diseases, probably due to their fiber, vitamins, minerals, and protective phytochemicals. It makes sense to get your children into the habit of eating whole grain foods now. Harvard researchers who studied the diets of more than 75,000 women for ten years found that women who ate more than two and a half servings of whole grain foods every day greatly reduced their heart disease risk as compared to women who ate no whole grains. How do you know a food contains whole grains? The label can help. Look for the health claim "Rich in Whole Grain."

How to serve: Give kids whole grain breakfast cereals instead of their highly processed, sugar-laden counterparts. Use whole grain breads for toast and sandwiches, serve whole grain crackers for snacks, and whip up a batch of oat bran muffins. Try brown rice instead of white, and encourage kids to try grains like quinoa, buckwheat, and barley as part of soups, stews, or side dishes. Serve whole wheat pasta. Add rolled oats to meat loaf. Serve popcorn to children over the age of four.

When to begin offering: As they get closer to their first birthday, your child can eat a wider variety of grains. Whole grains are fiber rich, so don't go overboard. Babies and toddlers can fill up fast on whole grains, leaving little room for higher-calorie foods. Small amounts of whole grains probably won't present a problem, however.

CHEESE

Why it's good for a growing body: Cheese is a protein-packed, calcium-laden food with near universal kid-appeal. It's also a source of vitamin B_{12} and the bone-building mineral phosphorus. Cheese comes in varying fat levels that can be used in a number of ways for a wide range of ages. For kids who eschew milk, cheese is a calcium alternative: 1½ ounces of hard cheese equals 8 ounces of milk in terms of calcium. The benefits of cheese don't stop at good nutrition. Research shows that eating cheese after a meal may actually thwart cavity formation by neutralizing the mouth acids that promote dental decay.

How to serve: You can serve up the goodness of cheese in any number of ways. Cheese can be part of an entree, a snack, or eaten as dessert. Kids love to nibble plain cheese, cheese and crackers, and melted cheese on toasted bread. Vegetables take on added appeal when cheese sauce tops them. Sprinkle grated cheese such as Parmesan on macaroni or on steamed vegetables. Kids can reap the goodness of cheese when it's used to make grilled cheese sandwiches, pizza, macaroni and cheese, and lasagna.

When to begin offering: Wait until eight months of age to serve your baby cheese, longer if your family is highly allergic (see Chapter 12, "Food Allergy and Intolerance"). Cut cheese into small pieces that tiny fingers can pick up and that children can chew with ease. Use milder-tasting hard cheeses at first, such as plain Havarti and mild cheddar.

YOGURT

Why it's good for a growing body: This versatile food is a kid-favorite. That's a good thing, since yogurt provides protein, carbohydrate, B vitamins, bone-building calcium and phosphorus, and zinc, which is helpful when your child doesn't eat enough meat products. Yogurt that contains live active cultures promotes intestinal health and boosts immunity, too.

How to serve: Children tend to go for highly sweetened yogurt with flashy packages, but you would do better to buy plain yogurt and sweeten it at home. Older children can decide on how to flavor their yogurt. Kids can add all-fruit preserves; fruit such as frozen berries or cubed fresh melon; dried fruit, including raisins and cranberries (but only if they are four or older); crunchy ready-to-eat cereal; molasses; or honey (no honey for kids under one year, however) to their plain yogurt. Chances are, they will use much less sugar than the typical 7 teaspoons that manufacturers add to 8 ounces of fruit-flavored yogurt. Yogurt-based fruit smoothies are fun for kids, as are dips made from yogurt. Plain yogurt tastes great atop a baked potato or sweet potato, too. As babies and young toddlers, Hayley and Hannah loved yogurt mixed with pureed fruit and thickened slightly with infant cereal. Emma loves full-fat yogurt mixed with peanut butter.

When to begin offering: Children can have yogurt at about eight months or so, later if there is a strong family history of allergies. Purchase full-fat yogurt with active cultures for children two and under, such as Stonyfield Farms' YoBaby brand. Give older children reduced-fat yogurts with live active cultures.

CHICKPEAS (A.K.A. GARBANZO BEANS)

Why they're good for a growing body: Chickpeas are packed with protein as well as the complex carbohydrates starch and fiber. They are also a source of iron, magnesium, folate, calcium, potassium, and zinc, as are many of their legume counterparts. In fact, kidney beans, lentils, and the like make suitable substitutes for chickpeas.

How to serve: Kids can be funny about legumes, rejecting them out of hand because of their shape or texture. Hannah will eat chickpeas just the way they are and as hummus, but Hayley prefers hummus only. No matter. Store-bought or homemade hummus is a kid-friendly food that can be used as a snack or turned into a meal. Try pita bread topped with hummus, and chopped melon for an easy lunch. My kids like lavash (roll-up bread) filled with hummus, too. For a snack, they dip pretzels into hummus. Try adding chickpeas to soups, salads, and pasta dishes. Puree chickpeas with chicken broth and use as a sauce on pasta or green vegetables. Add chickpeas to a vegetarian chili dish (but keep the seasonings mild to promote acceptance). Falafel may pique a child's interest in garbanzo beans because it uses the legume in a different way. A Middle Eastern favorite, falafel is a patty made from garbanzo beans that is easy to prepare at home.

When to begin offering: Babies can try mashed, plain garbanzo beans at eight months. Make sure to remove the thin skin around the bean before serving. To moisten, use a bit of chicken broth. Avoid serving heavily seasoned hummus to babies. Many commercially prepared varieties are loaded with garlic, so make your own when possible.

CANNED TUNA FISH

Why it's good for a growing body: Canned tuna fish harbors protein, vitamins B_{12}, B_6, and niacin, as well as small amounts of iron and zinc. While it's low in fat, the type of fat canned tuna fish contains is largely the omega-3 variety. Omega-3 fats are unsaturated fats with special protective properties. Often referred to as fish oils, omega-3 fats boost brain development and reduce the likelihood of heart disease in your child's future. Other, more oily, fish such as salmon and bluefish contain concentrations of omega-3 fats that beat tuna fish by a mile. But it pays to begin getting your child acquainted with seafood by serving milder-tasting seafood of any sort, since stronger flavors and odors can put kids off fish for a long time.

How to serve: Fish is an acquired taste for many American kids. A child may not be ready for grilled or smoked salmon (if they are, great) but willing to try a tuna salad sandwich. Try sneaking tuna into casseroles, too.

When to begin offering: Infants can try small pieces of moist canned tuna fish at about ten months or so.

Navigating Seafood Safety

Tuna fish garners attention for its potential mercury content. Canned tuna fish contains little, if any, of this potentially toxic heavy metal that can wreak havoc on the nervous system.

According to the FDA, the federal agency that oversees seafood safety, the larger species of tuna sold in stores and in restaurants as tuna steaks and as sushi contain about five times the mercury of canned tuna fish. Why the difference? Canned tuna is composed of smaller tuna types such as skipjack and albacore. In general, the smaller the fish, the less potential for mercury. Swordfish, shark, tilefish, and king mackerel—large, predatory fish—contain the most mercury. That's why the FDA advises pregnant and nursing women and women of childbearing age who may become pregnant to avoid these varieties of seafood.

BERRIES

Why they're good for a growing body: The likes of strawberries, blueberries, and raspberries are packed with carbohydrate, carotenoids, potassium, vitamin C, fiber, and disease-fighting phytochemicals. All that, with just a hint of fat and no cholesterol. To boot, this trio of berries ranks among the most powerful of fruits in thwarting cell damage that could result in chronic illness such as cancer and heart disease. Blueberries, strawberries, and raspberries supply anthocyanins, which appear to inhibit the production of cholesterol by the body, keeping arteries more clear. Proanthocyanin in blueberries is of particular interest for its ability to prevent a certain enzyme known for promoting cancer.

How to serve: Children love sweet, juicy berries and will eat them out of hand. Use berries instead of sugar to sweeten breakfast cereal; frozen may be substituted for fresh during the winter months. Concoct fruit smoothies with fresh or frozen berries. Layer with yogurt and crunchy cereal for a berry-filled parfait. Frozen or fresh whole or sliced berries and pureed berries make a healthy topping for frozen yogurt, ice cream, pancakes, waffles, and sponge or angel food cake. Add berries to pancakes, muffins, and other quick breads for their color and nutrition. Ditto for salads. Bake a fruit crisp or cobbler and serve instead of cookies for a sweet, nutritious treat. My kids love to dip whole strawberries in melted semisweet chocolate, and I'm sure yours will, too.

When to begin offering: Infants may eat berries beginning at eight months, but they should be well mashed or pureed to prevent choking. Wash berries thoroughly before serving.

BEEF

Why it's good for a growing body: Beef packs high-quality protein; vitamins B_{12}, B_6, and niacin; and the minerals zinc and iron in their most absorbable form. I chose beef over other meats because it's one of the most concentrated choline sources going. Choline is a B-like vitamin required for brain development and peak cognitive powers. In addition, beef contains the cholesterol and fat necessary for proper brain growth during the first two years of life. Lean cuts of beef contain the least fat and cholesterol and are the most appropriate for older children.

How to serve: Older children go for small amounts of ground beef as part of spaghetti sauce, tacos, and burritos, or as a burger.

When to begin offering: Infants may eat pureed, or finely chopped cooked ground beef beginning at eight months.

EGGS

Why they're good for a growing body: You can't beat eggs for top-notch nutrition, especially when it comes to protein. Eggs are considered the gold standard of protein quality because of their superior amino acid content. Egg protein provides all of the EAAs necessary to support life and growth. In fact, the protein eggs provide is so superior that all other foods are judged against the egg's amino acid makeup. Eggs are also the source for more than a dozen vitamins and minerals, and they are the most concentrated food source of choline, which is crucial for brain development in babies and in young children.

Now for the obvious question: Aren't eggs bad for you? Once considered cholesterol "bombs," a multitude of research has exonerated the egg, but parents still view it as a food to be avoided or strictly limited in family members' diets. Studies say that most people can eat an egg a day as part of a low-fat regimen without raising their heart disease risk. Despite their cholesterol count, which at 213 milligrams is admittedly high when compared to the recommended restriction of 300 milligrams a day, one medium egg supplies just 1.5 grams of saturated fat. Saturated fat is much more detrimental to health than dietary cholesterol. That's good news for parents and kids who enjoy this healthy food.

Above all, eggs are cheap, convenient, versatile, easy to prepare, and kids love them.

How to serve: You and your family can reap the many benefits of eggs in a variety of ways, including as omelets, quiches, and frittatas; and as part of waffles, crepes, pancakes, and French toast. Hard-boil a batch of eggs and keep in the refrigerator for up to a week for a quick snack, for egg salad sandwiches, or for adding to green salads.

When to begin offering: Babies may have cooked egg yolks at eight months, but wait until twelve months of age before giving them egg whites. Egg whites can be allergenic in children. Even so, chances are your child will have no problem tolerating the white of an egg. Serve infants chopped hard-boiled yolks or scrambled egg yolks (remove the whites and scramble for older family members or use in baking). Avoid egg substitutes in infants because they are made from egg whites only.

MILK

Why it's good for a growing body: Cow's milk contains calcium and phosphorus, two minerals critical for bone development and subsequent bone strength in growing children. Nearly all milk sold in the United States is fortified with vitamin D. Vitamin D regulates the body's uptake of calcium from food as well as bone calcium concentrations. In fact, getting adequate calcium without enough vitamin D does not ensure bone health and can certainly harm a child's chances of avoiding osteoporosis later in life.

In addition, milk supplies high-quality protein for growth and development and carbohydrate for energy. Full-fat milk provides fat and cholesterol for growing minds and bodies; reduced-fat milk is safe to feed your child after his second birthday. Milk is also a source of vitamin A and the mineral magnesium, which contributes to bone health. Magnesium may also be one of the components of dairy foods that research reveals helps to keep blood pressure in check. The Dietary Approaches to Hypertension Study (DASH) found that a low-fat diet rich in plant foods and three daily servings of reduced-fat dairy foods, including milk, lowered blood pressure as effectively as medication in adults.

How to serve: Most children love plain cold milk. Flavored milks, such as chocolate and strawberry, contain more sugar but no less calcium. Commercially prepared flavored milks may lack vitamin D, so read the label. Offer cereal with milk when kids won't drink a glass of milk straight up. Or make milk into a fruit smoothie or pudding. Prepare condensed soups such as tomato with milk instead of water.

When to begin offering: Aside from cow's-milk–based formulas, refrain from giving milk of any sort to your child until after her first birthday. The rationale for waiting to offer milk is covered in detail on page 88.

Chapter 11

Food Safety

for the

Entire Family

These days, there's a lot to consider when it comes to food safety. It's tough to figure out exactly what to look for when buying food.

—Hillary, *mother of three*

WHAT'S EATING YOU?

When your child feels sick to her stomach, it could be something she ate. According to the Centers for Disease Control and Prevention, Americans get sick from food 14 million times a year, and those are only the documented cases. Experts suspect that food makes people sick about 76 million times yearly. Why the discrepancy in the figures? Unless it's serious, foodborne illness tends to go largely unreported. People ignore it, chalking up their symptoms to the flu.

Everyone who eats is at risk for getting ill from consuming food contaminated with bacteria, viruses, parasites, and natural and manmade chemicals. Children, particularly infants, are even more vulnerable than adults to food contaminants because their immune systems and intestinal tracts are not as hardy. That's why it's more difficult for a youngster's body to fend off the germs that can cause health problems. Once foodborne illness takes hold, a child's system cannot battle it with the same intensity as an adult's can; kids with weak immune systems fare even worse. Diarrhea and vomiting, the most common effects of eating germ-laden food, are much harder on a little tike, in part because they lead to dehydration, which can have serious health implications. Your child's reaction to eating contaminated food depends on any number of factors, including the strength of his immune system, the health of his intestinal tract, the contaminant and its potency, and how much of the offending food he ate.

HOME FOOD SAFETY: IT'S IN YOUR HANDS

Most foodborne illness can be chalked up to bacteria found in animal foods. Viruses can be equally troublesome. They are simple organisms that require only food, moisture, and warmth to thrive to the point of wreaking havoc on your health. When bacteria such as *Staphylococcus aureus* (a.k.a. staph), or the Hepatitis A virus hitch a ride in foods held between 40°F and 140°F, these potential trouble-makers have all that they need to make you miserable.

Parasites are less common intruders, but they still pose a health threat. They can be found in raw meat and seafood. As a kid, you may remember your parents cooking your pork chops well done. They were trying to avoid trichinosis, a food-borne illness caused by parasites in pork. Trichinosis is much less common today due to diligent industry efforts to curb it.

Safe at the Plate

How much do you know about keeping food safe? Choose the best answer and see how you do. (And no looking ahead for the answers!)

1. The temperature of your home refrigerator should be:
   a. 50°F (10°C)
   b. 40°F or below
   c. I have no idea.

2. The last time you had leftover stew or any other meat, poultry, or fish dish, you:
   a. Cooled it at room temperature, then put it in the refrigerator.
   b. Put it in the refrigerator immediately after the food was cooked and served.
   c. Left it at room temperature overnight or longer.

3. The last time you handled uncooked meat, poultry, or seafood, you cleaned your hands in the following manner:
   a. Wiping them on a towel.
   b. Rinsing them under hot, cold, or warm water.
   c. Washing them with soap and warm water.

4. You defrost meat, poultry, and seafood in the following way:
   a. Set them on the kitchen counter until they are thawed.
   b. Take them out of the freezer and put them into the refrigerator.
   c. Microwave them.

5. You_____feed your baby directly from the jar of baby food.
   a. never
   b. always
   c. sometimes

Answers

1. **b**. Your refrigerator should always stay at 40°F or below. Measure the temperature with a reliable thermometer and adjust the thermostat if necessary. Check the temperature of your refrigerator periodically.
2. **b.** Refrigerate hot foods within two hours of cooking. If you leave them out for any longer, pitch them.
3. **c.** The only way to wash your hands is with warm soapy water for 20 seconds. Any other way doesn't kill germs. Dry hands with a clean towel.
4. **b and c are correct, but never answer a.** Keeping food out on the counter guarantees that germs will grow as the food warms up to room temperature.
5. **a.** Take a small amount of food out of a baby food jar and place in a bowl. Never return the uneaten portion to the jar for future feeding. Use a clean spoon to get more. Don't use the same spoon to feed baby.

How Did You Do?

Give yourself two points for each correct answer. Food safety is so important that if you scored less than 10, you must read on to learn how to correct your mistakes. Even if you got a perfect score, keep reading to find out more ways to protect your family from foodborne illness.

Outbreaks of illness caused by germs such as *Salmonella* and *E. coli* in foods including undercooked and raw poultry, eggs, and beef garner publicity, but lower profile organisms cause problems, too. For instance, strains of *Campylobacter* found in undercooked meat and poultry and in unpasteurized milk are the most common cause of diarrhea.

Food is an easy mark for germs, since it contains the prime conditions for growth: food, water, and warmth. Problem is, you cannot see, taste, or smell the elements of food bound to make you sick. Since no food is completely sterile, you should always treat it carefully when handling it and storing it. Here's how to keep food safe at home.

Shop Smart

Food should be in good condition before you toss it into your shopping cart. Check the expiration dates of dairy products, meat, and poultry. Refrigerated food should be cold to the touch, and frozen food should be rock-solid hard. Avoid canned goods with dents, cracks, or bulging lids—they indicate a serious food poisoning threat. Stay away from meat and poultry products with punctured plastic wrapping. After making a selection from the meat case, place it in a clear plastic bag. This will prevent any leakage of juices from the animal product onto other foods in your shopping cart. As for baby food, check to see that the safety button in the middle of the lid is down and that the jar is properly sealed. Even so, if the lid doesn't make a popping sound when opened at home, discard it immediately. Leave unpasteurized milk and juice on supermarket shelves, or at farm stands.

Bring It on Home

Shop last for cold foods such as meat and milk. Then go directly home and put them away. Never leave items such as milk, eggs, and poultry to sit in your car or in the trunk, which tends to be warmer than the rest of the car. If you must, store perishables in a cooler immediately after making your purchases. Take care, even when it's cold outside. Chances are, your car's interior registers well above the 40°F mark.

Wash Up

Frequent hand washing could cut by half the rate of foodborne illness and significantly reduce cases of cold and flu. Use warm water to lather up and wash carefully, especially before preparing food for yourself or your family. Always wash your hands after changing a diaper, visiting the bathroom, and handling pets. When working with raw animal foods such as chicken and seafood, wash your hands thoroughly before touching any other food, utensil, or any other surface, and before touching your child. Researchers at the University of Arizona have found that people had the most germs on their hands after making a meal, possibly because they failed to wash their hands after handling raw animal foods.

Be diligent with your youngster, too. Adults should stress the importance of washing up after every trip to the bathroom, before eating meals and snacks, and before helping you prepare food. Teach kids to wash for as long as it takes to sing the "Happy Birthday" song twice (about twenty seconds) while lathering up with warm soapy water. That's how long it takes to destroy most of the germs on your hands. Dry hands with disposable towels or a clean cloth, or air dry completely.

Is Food the Culprit?

Most types of food poisoning manifest themselves in the intestinal tract and are often characterized by vomiting and diarrhea. The sudden onset of intestinal problems without a cold, runny nose, cough, or body aches and pains should be enough to distinguish foodborne illness from the flu. In fact, it typically takes a day or so to develop the flu symptoms of fatigue and all-over achiness; this general malaise is usually accompanied by nasal or chest congestion, runny nose, cough, and fever. Depending on the germ, the symptoms of foodborne illness can be apparent in as little as thirty minutes.

When trying to determine if food is to blame when your child falls ill, it may be tough to get to the bottom of the situation, however. Youngsters don't always have the words to describe their discomfort or tell you what is going on in their bodies. It's even worse when trying to figure out how your infant is faring. Don't wait for a definitive answer. Call your doctor to discuss your child's situation. Make haste when children have any amount of bloody diarrhea, because it's a sign that your child may have consumed the potentially deadly *Escherichia coli (E. Coli)* O157:H7. The simultaneous symptoms of stiff neck, headache, and fever should be reported immediately, too. If your youngster vomits or has diarrhea two or more times daily for twenty-four to forty-eight hours, he may need to see his pediatrician, given his risk for dehydration and its complications.

Curb Cross-Contamination

You may be in for trouble when juices from raw meat, poultry, or seafood, or germs from unclean objects such as utensils, touch cooked or ready-to-eat foods. Separate raw meats and ready-to-eat foods such as salad greens. Make it easier to avoid cross-contamination by using separate plates for holding raw meat, poultry, and seafood and another for the cooked versions. When possible, designate separate cutting boards for raw animal products and for ready-to-eat foods such as bread and salad greens. Use different-colored boards so that you won't mix them up. Discard old cutting boards worn with cracks, crevices, and excessive knife scars because germs can thrive there.

Turn Up the Heat

Cooking destroys harmful bacteria, but only when it's done right. Animal products are particularly prone to foodborne illness, but applying the right temperature typically fends off troublesome germs. With the exception of eggs and fish, experts say that you cannot tell whether animal products are properly cooked by their appearance. Invest in a meat thermometer to be sure.

Here's what to strive for, temperature-wise.

- Whole poultry: 180°F
- Poultry breast and well-done meats: 170°F
- Stuffing, ground poultry, reheated leftovers: 165°F
- Medium meats, pork, and ground meats such as beef: 145°F
- Medium-rare beef steaks, roasts, veal, lamb: 145°F
- Egg dishes: 160° F. Cook egg yolks and whites until both are firm.
- Fish: Cook until the flesh is opaque and flakes easily with a fork.

Cool It

With all the outdoor partying going on, it's no surprise that a report from the Centers for Disease Control and Prevention cites the summer months as a time when foodborne illness caused by bacteria is at its peak. It doesn't have to be that way. To avoid getting sick from food, never leave it sitting out for more than two hours at room temperature, which is about 70°F. When the mercury climbs higher, food quality deteriorates even faster. That's why you should cool food after just one hour on the table. It's one thing to rely on your refrigerator and freezer for cooling, but you must make sure your refrigerator thermometer registers 40°F or below and that your freezer operates at 0°F or lower. If the units are any warmer than that, bacterial growth can occur. Also, don't pack your refrigerator or freezer with too much food. Cold air needs room to circulate in order to effectively squelch germ reproduction.

Mind the Marinating

When marinating meat, seafood, or poultry, use a covered plastic container and place it in the refrigerator. Marinade ingredients are acidic and cause a chemical reaction with some metallic containers that results in the metal leaching into your food. Never reuse marinade on raw animal foods such as meat, poultry, and seafood unless it's been boiled first to destroy any germs.

Defrosting Dilemma

It's so convenient to take out a package of poultry or beef and leave it to thaw on the kitchen countertop. But it is fraught with risk. As the food warms up at room temperature, germs begin to multiply. And although you cook it thoroughly, you may not be able to kill enough of the microorganisms to prevent foodborne illness. Here's what to do instead. Thaw food in the refrigerator; wrapped in plastic, sitting in cold water in a pan (change water frequently and refrigerate as soon as food is thawed); or in the microwave oven. Always marinate foods in the refrigerator, too.

Rhymes with Bacteria

Listeria. The name may be new to you, but food safety experts have known about this risky germ for decades. *Listeria monocytogenes* bacterial infections are on the rise in the United States. This hardy organism, which can grow even at cold temperatures and survive long bouts in the freezer, is causing more and more cases of foodborne illness.

Listeria monocytogenes bacteria cause a condition called listeriosis, characterized by flulike symptoms including fever and chills. Listeriosis may take from three to eight weeks to show up after eating contaminated food. According to the USDA, pregnant women and children are among those at greatest risk from *Listeria monocytogenes*. Moms-to-be can transmit the illness to their unborn babies, causing miscarriage, stillbirth, or other serious health problems. When recognized early on, listeriosis is treatable with antibiotics. However, it's best to do what you can to avoid listeria infections, since they cause nearly half of reported deaths due to foodborne disease. Most people don't get listeriosis, but of the ones who do, about a quarter of them die from it.

Intense heat, including pasteurization, is lethal for *Listeria monocytogenes*. Even certain cooked foods, including processed meats such as bologna and other lunch and deli meats and hot dogs, may be health hazards. They may become contaminated within processing plants or en route to your plate. *Listeria monocytogenes* may even be found in uncooked vegetables.

Avoid *Listeria monocytogenes* with these tips from the USDA:

- Reheat until steaming: hot dogs, luncheon meats, cold cuts, fermented and dry sausage, and other deli-style meats and poultry. If you cannot reheat these foods, do not feed them to children or pregnant women.
- Wash hands with warm soapy water for at least twenty seconds, and do the same for cutting boards, dishes, and utensils.
- Avoid unpasteurized dairy products of any sort. Soft cheeses such as Brie, Camembert, feta, and blue-veined or Mexican-style cheeses are particularly risky, but hard and processed cheeses, cottage cheese, yogurt, and cream cheese are not.
- Pitch foods that are past their expiration dates.
- Thoroughly heat all leftovers.

Don't Eat That! Foods Youngsters and Pregnant Women Should Avoid

Raw or undercooked animal foods, including eggs. They are the worst offenders as far as foodborne illness goes as they harbor a host of germs. Don't let your kids lick the batter bowl. The raw eggs used to make cakes, cookies, and brownies are risky for them and for you. Commercially prepared cookie dough is not hazardous, however. Neither are frozen desserts flavored with cookie dough or commercial products such as eggnog: they are produced with pasteurized eggs.

Soft cheeses. The likes of Brie, Camembert, feta, and blue-veined varieties of cheese may contain *Listeria monocytogenes*.

Unpasteurized juice and milk. Pasteurization kills nearly all the germs in juice and milk. It may seem more natural to serve unpasteurized juices or raw milk, but it is especially dangerous to feed them to a child or drink them when you're expecting. Unpasteurized juices must carry a warning label that states the dangers they pose, particularly to children, so read the package before purchasing or pouring.

Honey. Children under one year of age must avoid honey because of the threat of botulism.

Alfalfa sprouts. Animal foods are the usual vehicle for strains of the salmonella bacteria, but produce can be culpable, too. Alfalfa sprouts have caused outbreaks of salmonella poisoning affecting an estimated twenty thousand North Americans. Experts say that conditions are ripe for salmonella contamination in alfalfa sprouts given the circumstances of how the seeds are handled and then sprouted. And since consumers rarely cook or wash alfalfa sprouts, the chances of illness from eating them runs high. That's why alfalfa sprouts are frowned upon for people at the greatest risk for foodborne illness, including children and pregnant women.

Clean Up

Squeezing out a sponge doesn't rid it of germs, it just transfers many of them to your hands. Using dirty sponges or cloths also spreads microorganisms throughout the kitchen. If you prefer sponges, change them frequently and place them daily in the dishwasher to kill the bacteria they harbor. Microwaving a sponge for thirty seconds is also lethal for germs. Use a fresh paper towel to sop up each spill of meat, poultry, and seafood juice on countertops. Warm and cold rinses don't kill germs, which is why you should launder all kitchen towels and other cloths (as well as those used to clean the bathroom) in the hot cycle of your washing machine. For certain germ death, add bleach to the wash.

Problems with Plastics

Plastic is such a part of our lifestyle that you probably don't give it too much thought. You buy plastic-wrapped foods, store food in plastic, and even use it in the microwave. Plastics have pitfalls, however.

Plasticizers, used to make plastics pliable, are problematic because they can leach from wraps and bags into foods, including high-fat fare such as processed meats. The problem is that plastic degrades, causing chemicals to get into your food. Plastic's demise is accelerated by light and by heat; fattier and acidic foods absorb more plasticizers than other fare.

Some experts say that the plasticizer di-(2-ethylhexyle) adipate (DEHA), used in certain clingy plastic wraps designed for commercial use, is an endocrine disrupter. Endocrine disrupters are chemicals that can interfere with your child's development. Others, including the FDA and the EPA, say that studies have not confirmed that DEHA is an endocrine disrupter. While there's little scientific evidence to fear plastic, there's no reason why you can't handle it more safely. Here's how to avoid problems.

- Rewrap high-fat foods, including cold cuts, at home. Before eating, slice off a thin sliver where the commercial wrap came into contact with the food.
- Microwave foods in glass such as Corningware, or stick with brand names for microwavable plastics, including Tupperware and Rubbermaid.
- If you must use plastic wrap, purchase brands that specify on the label that they are made from polyethylene (such as Glad Wrap), because they don't contain DEHA. Leave a gap between food and any type of plastic wrap whenever possible.
- Store foods in glass, never in styrofoam.
- Never microwave food in leftover plastic containers such as cottage cheese or margarine tubs, and throw out old plastic containers that show signs of wear.
- Cover food with a paper towel instead of with plastic wrap when heating in the microwave.

(continued)

Consumers Union tested baby bottles made with polycarbonate, a clear, hard plastic material. When they filled them with infant formula and heated up the bottles, they found that bisphenol-A, a potential endocrine disrupter, leached into the formula. You could get around potential problems with plastic by using glass bottles. Another way to protect your baby: avoid clear, shiny plastic baby bottles and serve infant formula or breast milk in less shiny, opaque bottles, which are often colored.

IRRADIATION

The Food and Drug Administration (FDA) allows manufacturers to irradiate meat and poultry, fresh fruits and vegetables, and spices to reduce bacteria that can cause foodborne illness and spoilage, and to kill parasites and insects. How is food irradiated? It's packed in containers and moved by conveyor belt into shielded rooms. Then it's exposed to gamma rays or electron beams for a brief time. The process leaves the food essentially intact but is deadly for germs such as *E. Coli* O157:H7, *Campylobacter*, and *Salmonella*, some causes of foodborne illness. Irradiation can also put off ripening in certain fruits and vegetables and delay sprouting in the likes of potatoes and onions, thereby extending their shelf life.

Even with myriad benefits, irradiation is no substitute for safe handling of foods, including proper cooking and refrigeration. That's because it reduces the levels of germs but does not completely eliminate them.

The international symbol for irradiation, known as the radura, will tip you off that a food's been irradiated. The FDA also requires that irradiated foods state "treated with radiation," or "treated by irradiation." Irradiated foods are slightly more expensive. You may pay up to three cents more a pound for produce and upwards of a nickel extra for a pound of meat or poultry.

PESTICIDES

There's little doubt that the hundreds of different pesticides used on crops ensure a cheaper, steadier supply of produce because they maximize a farmer's yield. After all, pesticides repel any number of intruders that can damage crops, including insects and weeds. Without many of them, we'd be paying much higher prices at the supermarket with less variety to choose from.

Yet, no parent likes to think of his child consuming pesticides, given a child's delicate, developing body. What are the exact dangers of pesticides to a youngster's development? That's tough to say. The EPA says pesticides block the body's uptake of nutrients critical for proper growth and wreak havoc on development by permanently altering the way a child's system functions. Other experts go further, contending that pesticide consumption threatens the normal maturation of the nervous system, which could affect a child's physical coordination, memory, and learning ability. So far, scientists' concerns about pesticides are based on animal studies, however. That's why it's difficult to prove the effects of pesticides on humans.

Family Food Safety Rules
Never:

Refeed from same baby bottle, jar, or dish of baby food. When baby drinks from a bottle, mouth bacteria make their way into the milk and multiply. Ditto for a jar of baby food from which you have fed baby directly. The same principle applies to older children and adults, who should never drink directly from a milk, juice, or water container intended for later use by any family member. Refrain from eating directly out of peanut butter jars and ice cream containers, too.

Defrost breast milk on the kitchen countertop. No food should ever be defrosted on the kitchen counter. As the food warms, germs can multiply. Warm up frozen breast milk faster and with fewer consequences by immersing the bottle in warm water and swishing it around to mix up the fat.

Microwave a baby bottle of formula or breast milk. When it's 2 A.M., it's tempting to pop the baby bottle into the microwave to soothe a wailing child. But microwaving presents bigger problems, however. Uneven heating can make for hot liquid that can burn a baby's mouth.

Use ceramic dishes or lead crystal for food storage. Ceramic dishes and mugs, especially imported ones you've had for years, can be covered in a lead glaze. Lead from these dishes and from lead crystal decanters and the like can leach into food and hurt a baby's developing nervous system. Make sure your dishes are lead free with a home-testing lead kit available at hardware stores.

Even without scientific proof of harm from pesticides, consumer groups have a beef with the EPA's idea of what's safe for children to consume. They say that the government agency hasn't gone far enough to protect kids from harmful chemicals.

The Environmental Working Group (EWG) is one of the organizations that maintains kids are overexposed when it comes to pesticide residues in and on the foods young children consume most often. According to their research, more than a million American children ages five and under every day eat food that contains unsafe levels of thirteen pesticides collectively called organophosphates. Organophosphates are designed to disrupt the normal functioning of a pest's nervous system, effectively killing them off. The group estimates that of the 1.1 million children ingesting dangerous pesticide doses, 106,000 of them exceed the EPA's safe levels for *an adult* by ten times or more.

The EWG isn't the only organization to object to the EPA's pesticide limits for children. A report by a Committee of the National Research Council (NRC) concurs. *Pesticides in the Diets of Infants and Children* urges the government to develop new procedures for testing pesticide toxicity in youngsters, to collect detailed information about what kids eat, and to improve the methods of measuring pesticide residues in food. Most laboratory testing done by manufacturers to satisfy EPA requirements assesses pesticide toxicity in physically mature adults, according to the NRC. Among the report's other conclusions: some children could be consuming dangerous amounts of pesticides, and children may be more sensitive to the harmful effects of pesticides than adults.

Moving to Protect Youngsters

Under the 1996 Food Quality and Protection Act, designed in part to protect children in particular from the toxic effects of pesticides, the EPA is required to review the safety of about nine thousand existing pesticides in food. As a result of the new law, the EPA recently banned the use of chlorpyrifos, a member of the organophosphate family, from all domestic consumer products. Farmers may still spray crops with chlorpyrifos, but its use will be significantly reduced. The ban won't make for safer imported produce, however. Foods including New Zealand apples, Chilean grapes, and Mexican tomatoes contained the highest chlorpyrifos residues when tested by the USDA between 1994 and 1998, and there's no reason to think that will change any time soon.

After investigating the USDA's data on pesticide residues in twenty-seven thousand food samples, Consumers Union, the nonprofit group behind *Consumer Reports*, conducted its own study of risk. The group found that while the levels of pesticides on certain produce were within legal limits, they were not necessarily safe for children. To boot, some of the foods they have labeled most harmful— apples, pears, grapes, and peaches—are kid-favorites. It may come as a surprise that Consumers Union found imported produce no riskier overall than domestically grown fruits and vegetables. However, they did pinpoint specific imported fruits and vegetables that consistently contained high levels of pesticides: Chilean grapes, Canadian- and Mexican-grown carrots, Mexican broccoli and tomatoes, apple juice from Argentina and Hungary, and Brazilian orange juice all fared worse than their domestic counterparts.

A Pesticide Primer
- *Pesticide* refers to herbicides, fungicides, insecticides, and other substances that prevent, destroy, repel, or mitigate insects, rodents, weeds, fungi, and microorganisms such as bacteria and viruses. Pesticides also regulate plant growth, defoliate plants, and promote plant death.
- Since pesticides pose harm to pests, including animals and plants, they are, by definition, risky for humans, too.
- According to the EPA, about three hundred and fifty pesticides are used on our foods.
- Drinking water can contain pesticides when the chemicals make their way from nearby farmland to ground water or surface water systems that contribute to a drinking water supply.

Reduce Pesticide Exposure in Children
In spite of their findings that certain foods harbor harmful pesticides, Consumers Union does not recommend banishing fruits and vegetables from the diet. Even with pesticide use, the organization says that the health benefits of produce outweigh the risks from the pesticides they contain. Take the following steps to reduce your child's pesticide exposure:
- Choose foods with the least risk for harmful pesticides. According to Consumers Union, they include: frozen and canned corn, milk, domestic orange juice and broccoli, bananas, and canned peaches. Avoid riskier foods such as domestic and imported fresh peaches; frozen and fresh domestic winter squash; domestic and imported apples, grapes, spinach, and pears; and domestic green beans.
- Wash or peel all fruits and vegetables. Remove the outer leaves of leafy vegetables such as lettuce. Use products such as Fit Fruit and Vegetable Wash (Procter and Gamble) and Wash Dem Veggies (Vermont Soapworks) to remove water-resistant pesticides from produce.
- Eat a wide variety of foods to limit regular consumption of the same pesticide.
- Buy organic produce, particularly peaches, apples, grapes, pears, green

beans, winter squash, and spinach when you are able.

- Pesticides can be found in meat. When they are, they are most concentrated in the fatty part of the meat, so trim all visible fat and avoid eating poultry skin.
- Limit home pesticide use and never use products containing organophosphates and carbamates because they can interfere with your child's developing nervous system.
- Need an exterminator? Find one that practices integrated pest management (IPM) to tame unwanted pests.
- Check out pest control policies in your child's school or day care facility and urge them to use fewer pesticides.

What about Water?

Is your water safe to drink? Most likely, yes, unless your community is undergoing an outbreak because of contaminated water. Public water supplies contain the chemical chlorine, which, along with water filtration, reduces the levels of most harmful germs, with one exception: *Cryptosporidium parvum,* a chlorine-resistant organism, can make its way into tap water and cause illness in thousands of people at a time. Symptoms of *cryptosporidosis* include watery diarrhea, abdominal cramps, and fever. Children and pregnant women are among those at greater risk for cryptosporidosis. When outbreaks occur, boil your water for five minutes or purchase bottled water for drinking instead.

FOOD ADDITIVES

Pyridoxine hydrochloride. Niacinamide. Thiamin mononitrate. Sodium ascorbate. The gobbledygook on food label ingredient lists may sound suspicious, like chemical additives you want nothing to do with, never mind feed to your child. But wait. Pyridoxine hydrochloride, niacinamide, thiamin mononitrate, and sodium ascorbate are not toxic food additives, but beneficial ones. They are vitamins you're likely to find in your child's breakfast cereal. Luckily, not all of the nearly three thousand additives to food approved by the FDA are so hard to decipher. Household names such as salt and sugar are common additions to foods.

Food additives serve a number of purposes including keeping food fresh, boosting the appearance and flavor of food, increasing nutritional value, helping baked goods to rise, and fostering consistent flavor and texture. For example, the antioxidant nutrient beta-carotene provides margarine with its yellow hue; alginate, derived from seaweed, serves to maintain desired textures in dairy products; and alpha-tocopherol (a form of vitamin E) keeps the oils in foods fresher. Enrichment of foods replaces nutrients that are lost during processing, such as the B vitamins that are stripped away when milling flour for white bread. Fortified products provide nutrients not present in the original version of the food. For example, nearly all of the milk in the United States contains added vitamin D. And iron is often added to grain products to boost their nutrient profile.

In My Experience
Avoid These Additives

Not all food additives are suitable for children. Here are the ones that I avoid giving to my children and the reasons why.

Aspartame and saccharin. These low-calorie sugar substitutes are a boon for people with diabetes but essentially unnecessary for the rest of us, and for children. If your child needs artificially sweetened foods to keep his calorie intake under control, maybe he's eating too much. Give children the real thing in smaller amounts instead of artificially sweetened foods.

Nitrates and nitrites. These aditives are not safe. Plus, they're found in cured meats such as ham, bacon, and hot dogs, which offer little nutritional value and lots of sodium and fat.

Caffeine. A drug that causes little tikes to bounce off the wall. You don't need that from sugary soft drinks or bottled water, and neither does your child.

Olestra or Olean. A synthetic fat that provides no calories at all because it passes through the body undigested. In doing so, it takes with it beneficial carotenoids that may help prevent cancer and heart disease in your child decades later. So far, olestra is found primarily in snack chips, another food lacking nutritional merit. When my children have chips, they eat small servings of the high-fat variety.

While most additives are safe, many have pitfalls. Some, such as the sulfites used on produce and shellfish and in commercially produced bread products, can trigger allergic symptoms in certain people, especially those with asthma. Vegetarians who eschew animal products should know that some food components are derived from animals. For instant, the cochineal extract used as food coloring is extracted from the eggs of the cochineal beetle. Sodium nitrite is added to maintain the red color of cured meats including bacon, ham, and hot dogs. Sodium nitrite helps reduce the risk of the foodborne illness botulism, but it also forms potentially cancer-causing nitrosamines in your body.

ORGANIC FOOD: BACK TO BASICS

Organic refers to the way food is grown and processed. All agricultural organic foods must come from farms or processors certified by a state or private agency accredited by the USDA. Instead of conventional chemicals, organic farmers often use insects and crop rotation to control pests that damage crops. They also plant cover crops such as clover to add nutrients to the soil and reduce weeds, and they fertilize the land with compost and other organic matter. Livestock and poultry are raised without antibiotics or hormones. Still, organic foods may contain pesticides and other contaminants. The wind and water can carry contaminants from other fields, and the soil that farmers use to grow fruits and vegetables may contain pesticide residues, although probably very small amounts.

An *organic* label means food has been grown with minimal impact to the environment, which pleases some people. Others think organic food tastes better. Still others prefer it for their children because organic food is grown without conventional pesticides, and because it contains no artificial ingredients and preservatives. In addition, organic food is not irradiated or genetically modified. Organic foods are not necessarily more nutritious, however.

Right now, organic foods cost more than their conventional counterparts for a number of reasons: most organic food is produced by small farmers in small quantities; crop losses may be higher and yields may be smaller; and organic products must meet stricter regulations than conventional fare, a process that is often more labor intensive and costly. The good news is that as the demand for organic food increases, prices should gradually drop, making organic fare more affordable.

How does the government regulate organic food? The USDA sets the national standards for organic foods. Raw organic products are allowed to carry the USDA's organic seal if they are 100 percent organic. Processed products made from at least 95 percent organic ingredients could also tout the seal; those foods with at least 70 percent organic ingredients are labeled "made with organic ingredients."

BIOTECHNOLOGY BASICS

Genetically modified food is making a lot of headlines. More and more, we are eating foods that are genetically altered in some way, even if many consumers don't realize that modified foods can easily make their way into supermarket carts.

Breeding plants and animals for more desirable traits is nothing new. Hybridization, or interbreeding, is the traditional method used to improve the quality and quantity of crops. But even tried-and-true breeding techniques have their limits. For example, hybridization is time consuming and doesn't necessarily make for a plant with the best qualities. That's because hybrids contain all the genes of the parent plants, so undesirable aspects are part of the bargain, too.

Tinkering with genes allows breeders to select only the characteristics they want, and get quick results in the bargain. Transferring genes from one organism to another sounds scary and futuristic, but altering the natural order of things has its benefits. Using sophisticated techniques, scientists are able to insert gene fragments from bacteria or viruses into plants to make them resistant to disease. They can even move genes into other single-celled living organisms to produce life-saving medicine, including insulin. Scientists can also design plants that are resistant to pests and diseases, reducing the need for pesticides; increase crop production by developing hardier plants; and produce plants that yield healthier foods, such as cooking oil with less fat.

Thumbs Down to Genetic Modification

Gerber, Heinz, and Frito-Lay do not use genetically modified ingredients in their processed foods. Whole Foods Markets, owners of 107 stores nationwide, has also moved to eliminate foods from its shelves that are genetically altered or contain genetically altered ingredients, no mean feat.

So, what's the downside? The question of safety. Concerned consumers cite the fact that every day, we eat foods produced from transgenic crops without knowing about any of the long-term consequences. Some experts say that breeding "designer" crops will shrink the botanical gene pool, ultimately leaving plants more vulnerable to disease. Gene manipulation could dangerously elevate levels of naturally occurring toxins and allergens in plants, too.

Lack of labeling ranks high on the list of consumer concerns about genetically modified food. There is no way to tell whether raw food such as potatoes or tomatoes has been genetically altered, or if food products such as a muffin mix or baby food contain ingredients that have been, either. Some genetically altered foods such as soybean products are ubiquitous in the food supply; they are in everything from margarine to cake mixes. The FDA has proposed voluntary labels, but many consumer groups say that's not good enough.

You may want to steer clear of genetically modified foods, but it's probably next to impossible without mandatory labeling. Without a consistent labeling requirement, you won't know whether produce was grown with transgenic seeds or if a product is manufactured with genetically altered ingredients. The best way to avoid genetically altered foods is to buy certified organic foods. Organic certification prohibits the use of genetically modified organisms.

Chapter

Food Allergy
and Intolerance

People don't understand how scary it is to have a child with food allergies. My three-year-old son is allergic to milk, eggs, and peanuts. You have to be careful of foods that you can't even imagine would contain things that could hurt him.

—Colleen, *mother of two*

ALLERGY OR INTOLERANCE?

Confusion about food allergy and food intolerance leaves the door open for misinterpretation. You may think the terms are synonymous, making them interchangeable. Yet they are two very different conditions that require different approaches. Misunderstanding food allergy and food intolerance may lead to unnecessary dietary restriction. Read on to clear up the confusion.

ANATOMY OF AN ALLERGY

A food allergy, sometimes called food hypersensitivity, is a reaction mounted by your immune system to an allergen in food, which is almost always a protein. Your body mistakenly regards a harmless food protein as a threat to your body's wellbeing, and does what it can to repel it.

The first time you or your child consumes the allergen, it won't be readily apparent that the body is defending itself against the food's protein. There will be none of the myriad signs of food allergy, such as hives, swelling of the mouth and nose, or abdominal cramps. The second and third times around will be different, however. That's because after the initial encounter with an allergen, your body produced antibodies against it as a way to defend itself against subsequent "invasions."

Once the body has produced the antibodies to halt a particular allergen, you'll feel the effects of food allergy. After eating, the body releases massive amounts of histamine and other chemicals in response to allergens that trigger food allergy symptoms. According to the Food Allergy Network, it may take just seconds for an allergen to wreak havoc, but most likely the signs of food allergy appear within two hours. Sometimes it's a day or two before the allergen makes itself known with some of the symptoms listed below. Talk with your doctor if you or your child experience any of the following after eating:

- Abdominal pain and bloating
- Asthma or wheezing
- Chronic coughing
- Cramping
- Diarrhea
- Nasal congestion or runny nose
- Nausea
- Rashes (eczema)
- Shortness of breath

- Hives
- Itching and/or tightness in the throat
- Itchy eyes

- Sneezing
- Swelling of the lips, mouth, tongue, face, or throat
- Vomiting

Foods can produce many of the same symptoms without triggering an immune response. For instance, foodborne illness is culpable for diarrhea and vomiting, two signs of food allergy. Before you blame food allergy, your doctor must confirm that your immune system is involved, since this is the hallmark of food allergy.

Avoiding Anaphylaxis

Anaphylaxis or anaphylactic shock is a severe reaction to food—most commonly peanuts, tree nuts, fish, shellfish, and eggs—that can involve several parts of the body and any number of the symptoms of food allergy. The problem occurs when too many bodily reactions occur simultaneously, essentially overwhelming your system. As a result, blood pressure drops dangerously low and your heart may beat abnormally. Without treatment, anaphylactic reactions can be lethal. Children with asthma are at greater risk for fatal or near-fatal reactions from food.

ORAL ALLERGY SYNDROME

People with hay fever symptoms may also be allergic to certain raw fruits and vegetables, nuts, and seeds. The condition is called Oral Allergy Syndrome (OAS). OAS is caused by a cross-reaction of allergens in the pollen of birch, alder, hazel, grass, ragweed, mugwort, and in certain foods. Eating fresh fruits and vegetables can leave you with itchy or swollen lips, tongue, throat, or the roof of your mouth. OAS may be more irritating than life threatening, since it tends to cause problems in the mouth, lips, and throat, rather than all over the body. OAS symptoms disappear without treatment.

The following raw foods can produce OAS. Cooking typically destroys the allergens responsible for the condition.

- Apple
- Apricot
- Banana

- Honeydew
- Orange
- Parsley

- Carrot
- Cantaloupe
- Celery
- Cherry
- Fennel seed
- Hazelnut (filbert)

- Peach
- Pear
- Potato
- Sunflower seed
- Tomato
- Watermelon

FOCUS ON FOOD ALLERGY

In newborns and older infants who are allergic to the protein in cow's-milk-based infant formulas, the signs of food allergy will include diarrhea, vomiting, and a failure to grow properly. Your child may also bleed from his intestinal tract and be colicky. Switching to soy formula doesn't always remedy the situation, since many babies who are sensitive to cow's milk protein are also allergic to the protein in soy-based formulas and other soy products. If your child exhibits any of the symptoms mentioned in "Anatomy of an Allergy" on page 189, talk with your pediatrician immediately about the best course of action. Your baby may need a hydrosolate formula such as Nutramigen, Pregestimil, or Alimentum, or an amino acid infant formula such as Neocate or Neocate One+ brand.

As your child matures and you begin offering solid foods between four and six months of age, you may suspect certain foods are troublesome for your child. To get to the bottom of food allergies, keep a detailed log of what and how much your child eats, document the symptoms produced by each food, and how long the symptoms take to develop. If your child is cared for by someone other than yourself, have her track all the same particulars, too. Include vitamin and mineral supplements your child takes on the list. Don't rely on your memory to record what your child consumes. Write it down as soon as he's finished eating or drinking. Save labels from processed foods since they could contain ingredients that trigger food allergy.

Keeping a food diary is a step in the right direction, but don't try to manage food allergies on your own. Food allergy diagnosis requires a detailed medical history; physical exam; elimination diets that include avoiding the suspected foods; and, possibly, tests to rule out other conditions. Bring your child and his food log to a doctor who has intensive training in allergy and immunology for a full evaluation. Board-certified physicians who are allergy experts are reliable health professionals.

Diagnosing Food Allergy

Don't be too quick to diagnose a food allergy in your child, and don't let others be, either. Make sure that your board-certified physician conducts more than one of the following tests before confirming food allergy.

- Medical history
- Skin prick test
- Blood test
- Elimination diet
- Food challenge

Beware of the following tests; allergy experts say they have little, if any, scientific merit:

- Cytoxic blood test
- Sublingual provocation
- Intradermal provocation
- Food immune complex assay

Managing Food Allergy

There's only one way to manage food allergy and that's avoidance. Once you know which food triggers an immune response in you or your child, steer clear of it. Some children are so sensitive to allergens that getting a whiff of an offending food, or kissing someone eating a food with the offending allergen, can be potentially fatal. For instance, something as simple as sniffing the steam created by cooking fish can cause a reaction in fish-allergic people. That's why it's a good idea to avoid keeping foods that trigger allergy in the house, even if you have other children who can eat these products without consequence.

Keep It Healthy

There's a problem with avoiding foods with known allergens, however. In eliminating foods, you must amend your child's diet to make it adequate to fuel his rapid growth. Getting rid of milk because of an allergy means your child's calcium and vitamin D consumption will drop off to the point of jeopardizing bone development.

It becomes particularly difficult to manage your child's diet when she is allergic to more than one thing. Working with a registered dietitian (R.D.) can help, especially when your doctor recommends elimination diets and food challenges. An R.D. helps you to carry out the food restrictions your child must follow, while developing an eating plan that is tailored to your child's dietary needs. Find a registered dietitian in your area by contacting the American Dietetic Association. The organization offers a free, nationwide referral service.

Read Labels

Carefully reading food labels is critical for avoiding allergens. Depending on your child's allergy or allergies, there are dozens of offending ingredients you must avoid. The Food Allergy Network provides excellent label-reading resources. Still, food labels may sport unfamiliar ingredients; may not fully explain all ingredients; and manufacturers may change ingredients without warning, so don't take food labels for granted. One troubling labeling loophole: Manufacturers may list natural flavorings as an ingredient without spelling out their specific ingredients. Genetically modified foods pose a slight risk to highly allergenic individuals since the FDA doesn't require labels to state that foods include genetically modified ingredients. Some genetically modified foods may contain allergenic proteins from other foods that are not among the major allergens.

Before feeding processed foods with questionable ingredients to your child, call the company to clarify exactly what the product contains. When there is any doubt that a food is unsafe for any reason, don't buy it.

Curb Cross-Contamination

Watch for the warning "may contain . . ." on processed foods. Manufacturers add that statement to alert you to the potential risk of cross-contamination. Cross-contamination occurs when machinery used to make one type of food that doesn't contain potential allergens is then used to produce another product that could contain allergenic ingredients. When manufacturers fail to properly clean the equipment, cross-contamination can occur. For example, when tiny fragments of nuts make their way into a nut-free cereal, the person eating it is prone to an allergic reaction. The same is true for deli meats purchased at the supermarket. Cheese and deli meats, such as ham, that contain added casein, a milk protein, are often sliced with the same equipment used for other milk-free deli products.

Dining Out Dilemmas

Cross-contamination is also an issue in restaurants, making dining out with an allergic child no easy task. For example, French fries that are cooked in the same oil as fried fish are benign for most people but problematic for those hypersensitive to fish. Meat seared on the same grill as a tuna steak poses a similar problem.

Then there are the ingredients used to concoct restaurant foods. Nuts used in cheesecake crusts and pasta sauces such as pesto are potentially problematic; so, too, is the peanut butter or other "secret" ingredients used to thicken soups and sauces. And when the chef decides to get creative, watch out. One night Tom and I met friends for dinner at a local restaurant. Joe, who is allergic to nuts, ordered the same pork tenderloin dish as I did. Mine came first to the table. His entree arrived a minute or so later, looking slightly different. He was just about to take a bite when I realized the difference between the two meals: chopped nuts. Someone in the kitchen had garnished his meal with nuts. The kicker is that nuts were never mentioned in the description of the dish. If they had been, Joe would have steered clear of that entree.

Allergy experts advise extreme caution when eating away from home. To avoid hazardous dining-out situations, always ask the wait staff about the ingredients in restaurant food, and let them know what foods you or your child must avoid. If your waiter seems to lack confidence in his answers, ask him to query the chef about how the dish is prepared and to alert the chef to your needs. Many chefs will be as accommodating as possible. Stick to plain foods such as broiled chicken or steak, and avoid deep-fried and grilled foods. Try to dine out early in the evening (which is easy to do with kids) and stay away from restaurants on Friday and Saturday nights. This will help you get the special meal you need for you or your child with a minimum of mistakes and aggravation.

Top Allergenic Foods

Eight foods account for 90 percent of all allergic reactions, says the Food Allergy Network. Peanuts are the leading cause of food allergies, affecting about 3 million Americans. Overall, an estimated 6 to 7 million Americans suffer from one or more food allergies.

When feeding infants new foods, watch for any of the following food allergies. Introduce just one food at a time so that you can track your child's sensitivity. Feed that single new food for about five days, unless your child is bothered by it.

- Peanuts
- Tree nuts such as walnuts and pecans
- Shellfish, including shrimp, crab, and lobster
- Fish
- Eggs*
- Milk*
- Soy*
- Wheat*

*According to the American Dietetic Association, these allergies may disappear with time. Even though experts say cow's-milk allergy is the most common food allergy among children, kids tend to outgrow it by their fourth birthday.

At Day Care

Alert the staff at your child's day care center or kindergarten about his food allergy. Do what you can to educate them about your child's needs and about the importance of avoiding food allergy in general. A bit of planning can go a long way toward avoiding problems when your child is away from home.

Make a list of foods that provoke allergies in your child and write down emergency information about what to do when your child is negatively affected by food products. For example, not only is peanut butter problematic in the form of a sandwich, it can also be dangerous to a child with peanut allergies when used to make projects such as birdfeeders. Make sure all of his babysitters and teachers have the facts. Any medications your child needs should travel with him. A MedicAlert bracelet or necklace for your child is also a good idea.

Foiling Food Allergies in Children

If Mom, Dad, or both parents has a history of any type of allergy, including hay fever and asthma, it translates into a greater allergy risk for the children, including sensitivity to food.

The good news is that you can head off food allergies in children at risk. Avoiding allergies is based largely on delaying the introduction of the most offensive foods—peanuts, shellfish, fish, tree nuts, eggs, milk, soy, and wheat.

You can't change your baby's genetic tendency toward food allergies, but you may be able to minimize allergies. Try these tactics to reduce his chances of developing food allergies by following this advice from the American Dietetic Association and the American Academy of Pediatrics (AAP).

Breastfeed Your Baby

Among the myriad benefits of breast milk, putting off food allergy and reducing asthma risk ranks high. Breastfeeding provides the most protection against food allergies during the first three years of your child's life. Why? Breast milk bolsters your baby's immune system. It also provides your infant with antibodies that combine with potential allergens and prevent them from being absorbed into baby's bloodstream. By contrast, infant formula contains proteins that may be allergenic to your infant, especially when allergies run in the family. Breastfeeding moms of children prone to food allergies should eliminate all nuts, including peanuts (technically a legume); eggs; and milk from their diets. That's because the proteins from these foods can make their way intact into breast milk and cause problems in baby. Women who decide to eliminate milk need supplemental calcium and alternate protein and vitamin D sources, too.

Wait Until Six Months to Introduce Solid Foods

Experts say it's OK to give baby food at four months, but you should wait an extra two months to give your baby the edge on food allergy. This extra time allows your infant's intestinal tract to mature that much further. Here's the recommended schedule for more foods.

- Begin offering orange vegetables such as sweet potatoes and carrots at seven months. Wait five to seven days before trying a new food to see if baby is sensitive.
- Move on to green vegetables when baby tolerates the orange varieties. Serve up spinach, green beans, and peas. Read the labels of baby foods to avoid milk-based additives.
- Next, offer fruits, but only one at a time. Steer clear of products with potentially problematic additives including tapioca or food starch.
- At nine months, start giving baby grains and other vegetables such as oats, corn, and potato. Save wheat for last since it's allergenic in many people.
- Start adding meat at one year of age.
- Wait until your child's first birthday to offer cow's milk or soy beverages and products made from milk and soy.
- Hold off until two years of age to give eggs to your child.
- Steer clear of peanuts, tree nuts, fish, and shellfish until at least three years of age.

Looks Pretty, Tastes Good, Causes Problems

Artificial flavors and colors in processed foods can bother hypersensitive kids. Benzoic acid, sodium benzoate and tartrazine yellow, also known as FD&C yellow no. 5, can result in asthma and rashes; yellow no. 5 can be allergenic to people with aspirin sensitivity. Sulfites pose a hazard as well. They're used on a number of processed foods, including shrimp, and on certain fruits and vegetables. Sulfites can trigger asthma and anaphylactic shock in susceptible children and adults. Hydrolyzed vegetable protein contains monosodium glutamate (MSG), which has negative effects on certain people. Tragacanth is a gum that has resulted in some severe allergic reactions.

Make Iron-Fortified Rice Cereal Your Baby's First Solid Food

Stick with rice cereal for the first month, since it's less likely than other grains to be allergenic. Read labels carefully. Even single grain infant cereals may contain malt, which your baby should avoid early on.

Getting over It

Your child may outgrow food allergy. As a child's digestive tract matures, there is less absorption into the bloodstream of certain, but not all, allergens. A child's immune system becomes stronger with the passing years, allowing it to block antigens from wreaking havoc on the body, too.

There's a good chance that your child will outgrow allergies to milk, soy, eggs, and wheat. For example, after reaching age one, it's possible for children allergic to formula made from cow's milk or soy to be tested for their reaction to milk or soy beverages. But there is little likelihood that sensitivity to peanuts, tree nuts, fish, and shellfish will disappear with time.

How will you know when your son or daughter is old enough to try a food your doctor initially diagnosed as allergenic? Don't take it upon yourself to see whether your child has recovered from a food allergy. Discuss the possibilities of reintroduction with your pediatrician or allergist. Trying out the foods at home is dangerous for your child. And don't count on your doctor reintroducing foods that have in the past caused an anaphylactic reaction in your child, such as peanuts. You shouldn't, either.

ALLERGIES AND ASTHMA: WHAT'S THE CONNECTION?

Asthma is the chronic inflammation of the airways, which results in episodic wheezing, shortness of breath, tightness in the chest, and coughing that's more likely to occur at night and in the morning. It's the most common ongoing disease of childhood. Out of the 17.3 million Americans who have asthma, an estimated 4.8 million of them are children, according to the Centers for Disease Control. Asthma is on the rise in this country and worldwide.

The primary goal of asthma management is to reduce airway inflammation. Children who live with smokers and/or who are subjected repeatedly to other air pollution are more likely to have the symptoms of asthma. Sulfites and other food additives can trigger asthma attacks, as can food allergies. Youngsters with asthma and food allergies run a greater risk of having anaphylactic reactions.

FOCUS ON FOOD INTOLERANCE

Food intolerance does not involve the immune system, but it can be just as bothersome as a food allergy. Youngsters often outgrow food allergies, but a food intolerance may hang around forever. On the bright side, you may not have to completely eliminate "intolerable" foods as long as they don't also trigger allergic reactions. Food allergy and food intolerance can produce some of the same symptoms, so it may be difficult to differentiate the two when trying to figure out what's going on.

Milk Allergy

Milk protein is a common allergen in young children, yet milk allergies are actually quite rare in adults. That's because upwards of 85 percent of youngsters allergic to milk outgrow their sensitivity by the age of four.

If you think your child is allergic to milk, consult your doctor immediately. Removing all dairy foods and processed foods with milk-based ingredients without competent dietary advice is risky. Dairy products provide calories, protein, calcium, and a wide variety of vitamins and minerals essential to a young child's growth and development. Milk is the only dairy product that consistently provides vitamin D, which promotes strong bones by helping the body absorb calcium. Kids who cannot drink milk can count on fortified foods such as 100 percent fruit juice for calcium. However, despite their calcium content, these foods lack vitamin D. That's why you should work with a registered dietitian to plan a healthy diet for your youngster whenever food allergy is an issue.

Lactose Intolerance

Due to the absence of adequate lactase, people with lactose intolerance cannot properly break down lactose, the carbohydrate present in milk and other dairy foods. Lactase is the enzyme the small intestine makes to digest lactose. Symptoms ranging from mild gas to severe diarrhea that appear within minutes to hours after eating dairy products characterize the condition. Some people are so sensitive to lactose that they have trouble digesting processed foods that contain whey, casein, and whey protein concentrate, all of which contain small amounts of lactose. Certain medications even have a lactose base that makes them intolerable for some super-sensitive individuals. While the symptoms of lactose intolerance are uncomfortable, they pass within a few hours and are far less serious than those caused by milk allergy.

When it comes to lactose intolerance, quantity counts. Many people can tolerate small amounts of milk products without any side effects but become uncomfortable when they eat large quantities of cheese or ice cream, or drink lots of milk on an empty stomach.

Lactose intolerance ranks high on the list of common food intolerance in adults. When it comes to children, premature babies are at greater risk for lactose intolerance. An unborn baby's ability to process lactose develops during the third trimester. Since premature babies do not finish their term in utero, they are born with reduced lactase activity.

Looking for Lactose

Dairy foods are the most concentrated lactose sources, but they are not all created equal. Try smaller amounts of lower-lactose foods to avoid symptoms of lactose intolerance.

Food	Lactose (in grams)
Mozzarella cheese, part skim, 1 ounce	.08–.9
Cheddar cheese, sharp, 1 ounce	.4–.6
Ice cream, ½ cup	2–6
Cottage cheese, 1 cup	1.4–8
Yogurt, 1 cup	4–17
Milk, 8 ounces	9–14
Evaporated milk, 8 ounces	24–38
Sweetened condensed milk, 8 ounces	31–50

It's unlikely that your baby would have lactose intolerance if he or she was a full-term, healthy infant, but he could develop it with age. In fact, lactose intolerance is rare in African-Americans under the age of three and in Caucasians less than five years old.

A child of any age can develop a temporary form of lactose intolerance after intestinal infections. Youngsters who have conditions including chronic diarrhea may also be unable to properly break down the lactose found primarily in dairy products.

You or your child can still enjoy dairy foods even when you cannot tolerate lactose. Lactose-reduced foods such as Lactaid milk, Lactaid cottage cheese, and Lactaid ice cream are either free of lactose or contain minute amounts that won't produce stomach upset in nearly all lactose-sensitive people. Another option for reducing lactose in dairy foods is over-the-counter drops of the enzyme lactase that can be stirred into foods such as milk, cottage cheese, yogurt, and pudding. Tablets containing lactase can be consumed along with more solid foods such as pizza, lasagna, and ice cream to make them more tolerable.

Gluten Enteropathy

An inability to tolerate gluten is not common among children, but when it happens, it has serious repercussions.

Gluten enteropathy is the official name for a condition also known as celiac disease. In gluten enteropathy, the body cannot process gliadin, a part of the protein gluten, which is a constituent of many grains. When a child with gluten enteropathy consumes gluten, it damages the cells of the intestinal lining, which leads to inadequate nutrient absorption. As a result, the body does not properly absorb fat, carbohydrate, protein, vitamins, and minerals, and that leads to malnutrition. Weight loss and a failure to grow properly, nausea, and diarrhea are all hallmarks of gluten enteropathy. Children with gluten enteropathy run a significant risk of developing a host of medical problems, including abnormal bone formation and anemia, that could permanently affect their growth and development. Any child who has been diagnosed with gluten enteropathy should have a registered dietitian as part of her treatment team.

The treatment for gluten enteropathy is total avoidance of gluten, which would mean leaving out wheat, barley, oats, and rye products from the diet. Unfortunately, that's easier said than done, especially when it comes to processed foods. Many processed foods contain gluten in forms you wouldn't recognize. For example, modified food starch, vanilla extract, and vegetable protein all have gluten as an ingredient. However, several companies make many types of tasty gluten-free breads, pasta, and other grains that are suitable substitutes.

Chapter 13

Warding Off

Chronic Disease

I believe strongly that
what kids eat early in life
can affect their chances
of getting sick years later.
I try to keep my kids away
from foods that would
promote disease, including
ones rich in saturated and
trans fats, and produce
that's been treated with
pesticide. I don't always
do such a great job, but
I do make the effort.

—Alice, *mother of two boys*

With all the talk about the power of food, you are probably wondering how to best put food's preventative properties to work for your child. Maybe heart disease or diabetes runs in your family and you're eager to head it off early. Perhaps you want to do what you can to keep your child out of the dentist's chair or away from the doctor's office as much as possible. Maybe your son or daughter suffers from asthma and you're wondering whether there's a nutrition connection.

There is no question that most chronic illnesses plaguing American adults are linked to lifestyle; some have stronger documented connections to what we eat and drink than others. For instance, there's little doubt that most cases of heart disease are caused by poor health habits, while the connection between asthma and nutrition is just beginning to emerge.

Kids CATCH On

Just when you think your child isn't paying attention to nutrition advice, a study comes along to the contrary. Kids in grades three through five with access to healthful school lunches, well-designed physical education programs, and information about healthy habits ultimately improve their diet and increase physical activity for years afterward. That's the finding of the Child and Adolescent Trial for Cardiovascular Health (CATCH) study, the largest U.S. school-based health promotion program to date. Three years after the study was completed, researchers found that the then eleven-, twelve-, and thirteen-year-olds maintained a diet lower in total and saturated fat and continued to get regular vigorous physical activity without any outside coaching from adults. No doubt, parents who reinforce healthy habits taught in school-based programs would help kids stick to them for years afterward.

Healthy eating comes with no guarantees, however. Even the most exemplary diet cannot ward off all illness. Even so, there's no harm in helping your child develop healthy, lifelong eating patterns. Eating right could help prevent heart disease, stroke, diabetes, cancer, osteoporosis-related bone fractures, and birth defects in developing babies. Nutritious diets can also save money by reducing health care costs: The USDA estimates that better eating could save between $5.1 and $10.6 billion each year in medical costs, missed days at work, and premature death.

ASTHMA

Asthma is a chronic, potentially lethal lung disease. During an asthma attack, airways narrow due to inflammation, and breathing becomes difficult or impossible. Asthma is the most common chronic illness of childhood, and it shows no signs of abating. On the contrary, about 5 million American children suffer from asthma, which grew in prevalence by 72 percent from 1982 to 1994, according to the American Lung Association (ALA). Even more troubling is that more new asthma cases are diagnosed in children five and under than in any other age group.

Avoiding Asthma: Lifestyle Strategies

No one knows for sure why some children get asthma. Experts suspect that childhood asthma risk is partly hereditary and partly attributable to vulnerability to allergies. In fact, upwards of 80 percent of youngsters with asthma also suffer from allergies. Here are some steps to take to prevent asthma from affecting your child.

Don't smoke. Tobacco smoke puts kids at risk for developing asthma. In particular, children of smokers are more likely to develop asthma and to suffer from more asthma attacks, according to the ALA. Any smoker who spends time with your child should try to quit for their own health, as well as your son's well-being. In the meantime, don't let anyone smoke around your child, especially in a closed area such as a car, where fresh air is at a minimum.

Encourage weight control. Researchers have found an interesting connection between body weight and asthma risk in women and in children: Obesity increases the chances of developing asthma. In a study of nearly seventeen thousand children ages nine to fourteen years, scientists found that the most overweight children were up to three times more likely to develop asthma as the leanest study participants. The same researchers earlier looked at the relationship between obesity and asthma in adult women, and found that women became obese first, then developed breathing difficulties. As in the study conducted with children, the heavier the women, the greater the chance of asthma.

Encourage outdoor play. Breathing fresh air is one of the best tactics for warding off asthma in children. Yet, today, American children spend an unprecedented amount of time indoors, where they are subjected to a multitude of asthma-triggering substances, including dust mites, pet dander, cockroaches, dust, and mold.

Foster fish intake. The fattier the fish, the more protection it offers against asthma attacks, according to a study of Australian school children. The research, published in the *Medical Journal of Australia,* established a connection between regular consumption of fresh, oily fish such as Atlantic salmon, rainbow trout, and orange roughy and a reduced risk of asthma attacks. Can seafood keep asthma from developing? No one knows for certain, but experts say oily fish harbor omega-3 fatty acids that can reduce or prevent airway inflammation.

Pile on the produce. Some asthma experts believe that extra antioxidant vitamins such as vitamin C may protect against breathing difficulties. Vitamin C helps ward off the "oxidative stress" that can trigger asthma. Fruits and vegetables are the best sources of vitamin C, which may protect your child's airways. Plus, five daily servings of fruits and vegetables can help contribute to weight control that also wards off asthma. How? Produce is packed with fiber, helping kids feel fuller longer.

Make it a multivitamin. A daily multivitamin helps boost a child's immunity by providing nutrients he may miss out on in food.

CANCER

Cancer is characterized by unchecked growth of abnormal cells. In adults, years of damage to the genes in your cells trigger the out-of-control spread of unhealthy tissue that can invade other parts of the body and possibly result in death. Among American adults, cancer is second only to cardiovascular disease as the leading cause of death.

Anyone can get cancer, but some are more likely than others. Age plays a role. About 80 percent of cancer is diagnosed in people fifty-five or older. That makes sense, given that the older you are, the greater your exposure to the carcinogens (cancer starters) that can damage cells, including chemicals, radiation, smog, viruses, and hormones.

Childhood cancers are rare and differ from cancers diagnosed in adults. Children are more vulnerable than adults to leukemia, bone cancers, and cancer of the brain and other parts of the nervous system, while the leading cancers in adults include skin, prostate, breast, lung, and colorectal tumors. The reasons for most of the childhood cancers are unknown, yet experts say that unlike most cancers in adults, childhood cancers are not significantly related to years of poor health habits such as an unhealthy diet or sedentary lifestyle.

Curbing Cancer: More Than Just Diet

Genetics plays a role in cancer development, but family history cannot fully explain cancer risk, says the American Cancer Society (ACS). Upwards of a third of all cancer deaths are related to a poor diet; even more are linked to unhealthy habits such as smoking cigarettes. A healthy lifestyle can make a dent in cancer risk. Eating right, staying physically active, and maintaining a healthy weight from childhood on can cut chances of adult cancer by 60 to 70 percent, according to the American Institute for Cancer Research.

Don't get fired up. It's not just what you eat, it's how you prepare it that counts when curbing cancer. Grilling meat, poultry, and seafood may actually promote cell damage that leads to tumors. High heat produces heterocyclic amines, or HCAs, which scientists say may cause cancer in humans. Meat and poultry lead the pack in HCA production when grilled, while seafood supplies far fewer of the detrimental chemicals. Fruits and vegetables produce few, or no, HCAs when grilled. Other high-heat cooking methods threaten health, too. For example, broiling and pan-frying meats generate far more HCAs than baking or roasting.

Polycyclic aromatic hydrocarbons, or PAHs, form when the fat from foods comes into contact with a flame, heating element, or hot coals. PAHs float up in the smoke and plop themselves onto your child's food. PAHs may also form directly on food when it's cooked to a crisp.

For Adults Only

In its report, *Food, Nutrition and the Prevention of Cancer: A Global Perspective*, the American Institute for Cancer Research recommends total alcohol avoidance as one of their many dietary measures to thwart cancer. If you drink, limit alcohol consumption to less than two drinks daily for men and one a day for women.

If your family loves grilled meat, try using lower fat cuts. They contain less fat and produce fewer PAHs. Decrease cooking time by thawing frozen meat, poultry, or seafood first to reduce exposure to cooking elements, and precooking meats so that they spend less time on the grill. Cut meat and poultry into smaller pieces to cook more quickly (skewered kabobs cook the fastest). Trim fat from meat and remove skin from poultry before cooking. Grill seafood more often than meats. Fish tends to contain less fat, which means fewer PAHs.

Grilled vegetables and fruits, and veggie or tofu burgers, produce few, if any, potential carcinogens. Fruit, including pineapple chunks, peaches, and pears, may be skewered and broiled directly or wrapped in foil and grilled for a sweet and refreshing side dish, appetizer, or dessert.

Avoid processed meats. Ham, frankfurters, bacon, and sausages contain added nitrites to prevent spoilage and preserve color. Once your child consumes nitrites, they are converted in the stomach to nitrosamines, which are potent carcinogens, or cancer starters. If your youngster must consume processed meats, make sure to serve them with foods or beverages rich in vitamin C. Vitamin C helps thwart the formation of nitrosamines.

Pile on the plant foods. Scientific scrutiny of populations who eat the most servings of fruits and vegetables points to the protective effects of produce. It seems that on the whole, the groups of people consuming the greatest amount of fruits and vegetables run the lowest risk for developing cancers of the skin, lung, cervix, esophagus, stomach, colon, pancreas, breast, and prostate. The American Institute for Cancer Research recommends a predominantly plant-based diet rich in a variety of fruits and vegetables, legumes (includes chickpeas, lentils, and other beans), and whole grains. Encourage kids to eat at least five servings of fruits and vegetables every day.

Stay Away from My DNA

There are dozens of different cancer types, but they all have something in common: DNA damage. DNA is the cell's blueprint for reproduction. Genes are a part of the DNA in every cell in your body. Mutations to the genes that regulate cell growth spell trouble because they cause cells to make defective copies of themselves and proliferate out of control. Cancer takes years to develop in adults. According to the American Cancer Society, a decade or more may go by between exposure to carcinogens and cancer detection in the body. The trick in preventing cancer is warding off cell damage, which can be largely achieved through a healthy lifestyle, including eating right.

Get a move on. Daily physical activity reduces cancer risk and it fosters a healthy weight. A study conducted at the University of Southern California at Los Angeles found that premenopausal women who exercised moderately for three hours a week lowered their breast cancer risk by 30 percent; women who worked out four or more hours a week were 50 percent less likely to get breast cancer. Try to exercise with your children at least five times a week.

Snuff out smoking. Kids are under a lot of pressure from their peers to try smoking, but they still look to their parents as the ultimate role models. Even if you smoke, you probably don't want the same for your child. That's why you should try to quit immediately. Smoking increases your chances of cancers of the mouth, lungs, throat, larynx, bladder, and other organs. According to the ACS, the estimated 173,000 cancer deaths from smoking in 1999 could have been avoided.

Fight flab. Being overweight or underweight during adulthood boosts the threat of cancer. Help your kids achieve and maintain a healthy body weight during childhood to decrease cancer risk later on.

Slather on the sunscreen. Exposure to sunlight is cumulative. Sunburns during childhood increase the risk of skin cancer as an adult. The majority of skin cancers could be prevented by proper protection from strong sunlight, which includes covering kids in sunscreen with a protective factor of 15 or above. Set a good example by wearing sunscreen yourself, covering up at the beach, and wearing a hat that shades your face. Do not use sunscreen on infants six months and younger. Keep them covered and in the shade instead.

CARDIOVASCULAR DISEASE

Despite its decline, cardiovascular disease kills more American adults than any other condition. High blood pressure and coronary heart disease are the predominant forms of cardiovascular disease, although stroke or "brain attack" falls into the category, too. It's possible to have more than one form of cardiovascular disease, and it's more than likely that as you age, you will.

Heart Disease Alert

Risk factors for coronary heart disease include: family history; being male; low blood levels of high-density lipoprotein (HDL), the "good" cholesterol; elevated blood cholesterol level; high blood pressure; cigarette smoking; elevated blood glucose levels such as those seen in diabetes; inactivity; and high concentrations of triglycerides (fat) in the blood.

Coronary heart disease is caused by atherosclerosis, the slow and steady narrowing of the coronary arteries, the large blood vessels that ferry oxygen-rich blood to the heart and the brain. Plaque buildup on the lining of the artery walls is the hallmark of atherosclerosis. Problems with plaque arise when the buildup chokes off the blood supply and leads to tissue death. When that happens in arteries that supply the heart, it's called a heart attack; when it affects the brain, it's called a stroke or "brain attack."

Cut Cardiovascular Disease Risk: Lifestyle Strategies

Control blood cholesterol levels. There is a strong connection between the risk of coronary heart disease and elevated blood cholesterol concentrations. Furthermore, scientific studies conducted on teenagers killed in accidents confirm the relationship between plaque development in their arteries and elevated levels of low-density lipoprotein (LDL), the "bad" cholesterol, in the bloodstream. LDL, which is formed in the liver, is the transport vehicle for the majority of cholesterol in the body. The higher the LDL, the greater the risk of heart disease.

Kids and Cholesterol

Should you be concerned about you child's cholesterol level? That depends. Not every child requires a blood test. Here's who needs to be aware of their blood cholesterol concentration: Youngsters with a parent or grandparent who has suffered a heart attack or stroke, or who has been diagnosed with peripheral vascular disease or any other cardiovascular disease harmful to the blood vessels before age fifty-five; kids with one or more parent with a blood cholesterol reading of 240 milligrams/deciliter (100 milliliters of blood) or higher; and adopted children.

One elevated cholesterol reading does not make for a risk factor. Have your doctor confirm your youngster's initial test results two weeks later before concluding that your son has a cholesterol problem.

Here's the scoop for children two and older.

Category	Total Cholesterol (milligrams/deciliter)	LDL Cholesterol (milligrams/deciliter)
Acceptable	less than 170	less than 110
Borderline	170–199	110–129
High	200 or greater	130 or greater

Source: The National Cholesterol Education Program's Expert Panel on Blood Cholesterol in Children and Adolescents

---

If your doctor diagnoses your child with elevated blood cholesterol, dietary therapy will be tried first to normalize the levels. Your pediatrician may recommend a low-fat diet (less than 30 percent fat calories) as well as a reduction in saturated fat intake. Just a few meetings with a registered dietitian can help you better understand the many dietary recommendations needed to curb blood cholesterol in a child over the age of two.

From about age two, you may gradually begin reducing the total and saturated fat in your youngster's diet, but there's no reason to severely restrict fat in an effort to get a leg up on atherosclerosis if your child has no documented heart disease risk factors. The goal for fat intake is 30 percent or fewer calories from fat by the age of five. You have plenty of time to meet this dietary goal, so don't rush it. Cutting back on fat could limit a very young child's growth and brain development. Instead, encourage variety, and work in fiber as your child matures. Fiber helps fight off elevated cholesterol as one of its many benefits (see "Fiber," page 16). Never restrict fat intake in a child under the age of two, unless a medical condition dictates it for some reason.

Stop cigarette smoking before it starts. Smoking increases the risk of atherosclerosis and stroke. The AAP recommends educating kids about the dangers of smoking beginning early in life. If you smoke, try to quit for your sake, and for your child's.

Encourage regular physical activity. Regular physical activity makes the heart strong, keeps blood cholesterol in check, and fosters weight control, among its myriad benefits to the entire body and mind. In addition, physical activity boosts levels of HDL, the beneficial type of cholesterol that's connected to a lower risk for heart disease in adults.

Identify and treat high blood pressure. Elevated blood pressure increases the risk of heart attack and stroke. A certain number of children inherit high blood pressure without any apparent risk factors. Overweight children run a greater risk for high blood pressure. Even in children as young as two, being overweight can elevate blood pressure.

Avoid becoming overweight. Overweight youngsters are more likely to be overweight adults, setting the stage for certain cardiovascular disease. In fact, obesity alone is associated with early atherosclerosis in young adults, even when it's independent of other risk factors for the disease. Carrying around extra body fat taxes the heart muscle and increases the likelihood of elevated blood cholesterol levels that could lead to clogged arteries. If your pediatrician determines your child is overweight, begin making dietary changes (see "Overweight and Obesity," page 222 for more details). The typical treatment for overweight kids is to wait for them to grow taller while preventing additional fat gain.

Treat diabetes. Uncontrolled diabetes in kids and adults damages blood vessels, including the arteries that lead to the heart and the brain. In fact, people with diabetes are two to four times as likely to suffer from heart disease and just as likely to have a stroke, according to the American Diabetes Association. If your child has been diagnosed with diabetes, make every effort to keep blood glucose levels within the ranges suggested by your doctor.

Fight with folate. Folate and folic acid reduce levels of homocysteine, an amino acid associated with clogged arteries in adults.

Serve up soy. Soy protein reduces blood cholesterol levels. Tofu, tempeh, roasted soy nuts, and soy beverages are particularly good sources.

How Plants Can Help Hinder Heart Disease

Plant foods contain naturally occurring compounds called phytochemicals. Flavonoids are but one group of phytochemicals that your child can benefit from. In population studies, high intakes of flavonoids were associated with a lower risk of coronary heart disease. How do phytochemicals such as flavonoids work to ward off heart disease? No one knows for sure, but experts say phytochemicals' effects are twofold: they prevent the conversion of LDL-cholesterol to a stickier form that's more likely to clog arteries and they reduce the ability of passing red blood cells to clump and adhere to accumulating plaque within the arterial wall. Luckily, flavonoids are abundant in kid-friendly foods, including berries, cherries, grapes, apples, whole grains, grapefruit and grapefruit juice, and broccoli.

DENTAL CARIES (CAVITIES)

Dental caries is a fancy term for cavities, which can be a real pain, both physically (for your child) and financially (for you). Cavities are the number one cause of tooth loss in the United States, according to the American Dental Association (ADA). Thanks largely to fluoride, dental caries are on the decline in this country, but they remain a major problem in adults and children. Thirty percent of all kids develop some type of cavity from age five to seventeen. As children mature, the rate of tooth decay increases: two- to six-year-olds have half the decay of twelve- to seventeen-year olds. Tooth decay in early life leaves teeth weaker and more likely to pose dental problems later on.

How do cavities happen? Blame it on bacteria. Within minutes after eating, the germs that live in your mouth begin gobbling up the simple sugars and starch left there by food and form plaque. As they munch, plaque bacteria create acid that annihilates enamel, the tooth's hard outer protection. Mouth bacteria thrive on the carbohydrate contained in both the healthy and the not-so-nutritious foods kids consume, including dairy products, fruit juice, candy, grains, and sugary soft drinks. After many battles with acid, a tooth may succumb to decay, and you have yourself a cavity.

Some children are more susceptible than others to cavities. In fact, surveys show that just 25 percent of children ages five to seventeen harbor 80 percent of all cavities. What's the reason? Genetics may play a role. Some people have fewer cavity-causing germs in their mouths than others. Parents and other caregivers can transmit detrimental mouth bacteria to their little loved ones, too. Studies suggest that high concentrations of harmful mouth bacteria in Mom makes for a greater risk of cavity-causing bacteria in her child.

Whatever the case, a healthy diet and stellar dental hygiene help halt cavity formation. Brushing teeth twice daily with a fluoride toothpaste that has the American Dental Association Seal of Acceptance, daily flossing, and regular dental checkups can help defeat problematic plaque buildup.

Dodging Dental Caries: Strategies for Success

A healthy diet is one of the best defenses against dental disease, including cavities. Getting adequate nutrients over a long period of time is paramount for forming hard teeth and healthy gums that can repel the effects of acid-producing bacteria. A well-balanced diet also bolsters your youngster's immune system, which thwarts potential damage from germs. Here's what it takes to eat for dental health.

More than slime. Saliva prevents bacteria from adhering to teeth; speeds clearance of carbohydrate from your mouth after eating; and contains protective elements, including the immunoglobulins that depress bacterial growth. Chewing sugarless gum stimulates saliva production, especially helpful when kids cannot brush their teeth. Don't give gum to children under the age of four, or to youngsters over four who cannot understand the importance of not swallowing it.

Milk makes might. Children two and older require at least two servings a day from the dairy group. Dairy foods are rich in calcium and phosphorus, two minerals you must have to form teeth and bones and keep them strong. Milk is particularly beneficial for dental health because it's the only dairy product that consistently contains added vitamin D. Vitamin D is necessary for calcium absorption and deposition into the teeth and the bones that support and hold teeth in place. Plant foods, including dark green leafy vegetables and figs, provide valuable amounts of calcium, as do calcium-fortified orange juice and tofu processed with calcium sulfate, but they don't provide kids with the vitamin D they need. Children with milk allergies or who otherwise avoid milk probably need supplemental vitamin D. A daily multivitamin designed for children should suffice.

C for collagen. Vitamin C is a vital component of collagen, the connective tissue found in teeth and bones. It is also necessary for gum health. Inadequate vitamin C may translate into bleeding and swollen gums, which increases the risk for tooth decay and tooth loss. Offer your child at least one daily serving of produce rich in vitamin C, including oranges, kiwi, strawberry, and tomato.

Focus on fluoride. Fluoride toughens tooth enamel, making it harder and more resistant to decay. Fluoride works in two ways. As part of toothpaste, mouth rinses, fluoridated water, and professionally applied gels and rinses, fluoride gets incorporated into the surface of the tooth, bolstering strength. When swallowed as part of fluids, foods, or supplements, fluoride becomes an integral part of forming teeth, getting evenly distributed throughout the entire structure, which further increases a tooth's resistance to acid from mouth bacteria. Fluoride's protective effect is greatest when given during the time of peak tooth formation, including before teeth become visible to the naked eye, according to the National Research Council (NRC). The fluoride you swallow is also incorporated into the saliva that bathes teeth, helping to keep cavities at bay.

Caring for Baby's Teeth

Your infant was born with a full set of teeth just waiting to erupt, and you want to ensure that he goes through life with all of them intact. Even though you cannot detect any teeth coming through his gum tissue, it's never too early to begin caring for his dental health. Baby teeth mark the space in the jaw for when the adult teeth come in. Losing a baby tooth to decay early on may mean the teeth on either side move into the empty space. That makes for crooked or crowded teeth once your child's secondary teeth appear. Until he cuts his first tooth, gently wipe your baby's gums after every meal or snack with a soft, damp cloth to rid his mouth of harmful bacteria. Once teeth appear, brush them twice a day with a fluoride toothpaste.

Give the slip to sticky snacks. The longer a food or drink lingers in your mouth, the more harmful to teeth. Stickier foods such as white bread, pretzels, snack chips, crackers, and cereal are among the worst for teeth. Add sugar to the mix, and the threat of cavities increases. That's why cookies and muffins rank as even worse offenders. Cheese is a different story, however. Nibbling on a small wedge of aged cheese such as cheddar after meals or instead of high-carbohydrate snacks provides a triple threat to mouth bacteria: Cheese deprives plaque of a food source, it provides teeth and bones with calcium to help them to stay strong, and cheese neutralizes the harmful acids created by mouth germs. In addition, the fat in cheese is actually beneficial for teeth because it speeds up clearance of lingering carbohydrate from the mouth.

Banish the bottle. Children ages three and under are the most likely to suffer from baby bottle tooth decay, destruction that occurs primarily in the upper front teeth. Youngsters who are allowed unlimited access to milk, juice, and other sugary soft drinks are prone to baby bottle tooth decay, even when they drink from a "sippy" cup. The carbohydrate contained in these beverages bath the teeth, providing a constant food source for plaque bacteria. This results in rampant tooth decay, which is not always confined to the front of the mouth. It seems strange, but breastfed babies can also be victims of "baby bottle" tooth decay when their teeth are exposed to breast milk for too long. Prevent tooth decay in your infant and toddler with these suggestions: Never put a baby to sleep with a bottle if you cannot clean his teeth after he drinks, offer beverages in a cup, discourage access to sugary drinks, and never fill your child's bottle with juice or soda of any type. Don't use a bottle as a pacifier to soothe a fussy baby, and avoid offering your child a pacifier dipped in any sweet liquid or in sugar. Wipe your baby's gums with a clean damp soft washcloth after every feeding. Remove your breastfed baby from the breast as soon as he is done eating.

Check it out. Plaque begins forming at about six months of age, so a child's dental problems can easily begin during infancy. Don't wait until your child has a mouth full of teeth to visit the dentist. Take children to the dentist by their first birthday to better spot any problems that could plague them for the rest of their lives. Regular dental checkups and guidance from your dentist during childhood are particularly critical since enamel formation is nearly complete by the time a youngster enters first grade. Seeing a dentist early and often can put off decay in other ways, too. For example, your dentist may advise sealants for your child's teeth. Sealants are applied to the chewing surfaces of a child's back teeth, acting as a barrier from acid-producing bacteria.

Brush it off. Each time your child eat sugars or starches, acid from mouth bacteria attack your teeth for at least twenty minutes, according to the American Dental Association. That's why you shouldn't allow food to stick around in your child's mouth. It may be difficult, but try to get kids into the habit of brushing their teeth twice a day with fluoride toothpaste. Monitor the amount of tooth-paste they put on their brush, as they need just a dab no bigger than a pea. Make sure kids brush after they eat or drink anything other than water at night before going to bed. Kids ages four and five can brush their teeth by themselves, but you should check to see if they have reached all areas of their mouth. Start flossing your child's teeth when two of his teeth begin to touch. When kids can't brush, have them swish and rinse with water, or drink water to wash away carbohydrate; older children can do the same by chewing sugarless gum.

Get a Jump on Gingivitis

Gum diseases, such as gingivitis, don't often come to mind when considering your child's dental health. Yet, according to the American Academy of Pediatric Dentistry, studies suggest that about half of all children ages two and three have at least mild inflammation of their gum tissues, one of the signs of gingivitis. The problem may be worse in their parents. About 75 percent of Americans over the age of thirty-five suffer from some form of gum disease, which can lead to tooth loss.

Gingivitis is the typically painless, early stage of periodontal disease that affects the gums only. Periodontal disease is a general term for the bacterial infections that affect the area surrounding the tooth, including gums, ligaments (connective tissue), and the bone that anchors teeth.

As in the case of cavities, mouth bacteria are to blame. Brushing daily reduces plaque buildup, but may not completely remove it, particularly around the gum line. That's why flossing teeth every day is so important. Lingering plaque forms a rough, porous material called tartar, the stuff dental hygienists scrape off during a checkup and cleaning.

The good news is that gingivitis can be stopped. Brushing twice a day, cleaning between teeth, and regular dental cleanings can reverse gingivitis and prevent it from turning into periodontitis, advanced gum disease. Periodontitis destroys the tissues that secure teeth to bone, promoting tooth and bone loss. The condition exposes the roots of teeth to bacterial toxins by fostering the formation of pockets that make teeth vulnerable to decay and sensitive to cold foods and beverages and to touch. Watch for these telltale signs of gingivitis and periodontal disease:

- Gums that bleed easily
- Red, swollen, or tender gum tissue
- Gum tissue that has pulled away from the teeth
- Pus that oozes from between the teeth and gums when pressure is applied to gums
- Persistent bad breath or bad taste in your mouth
- Permanent teeth that are loose or separating
- Any change in the way your teeth fit together when you bite
- Any changes in the fit of partial dentures

Timing is everything. High carbohydrate foods such as refined, low-fiber cereals, white bread, and juice are harmful to teeth when eaten alone, but when taken along with balanced meals, they aren't as detrimental. Combining carbohydrates with protein-rich foods such as nuts, hard cheeses like cheddar and Swiss, eggs, and meat limits detrimental acid production. Why? Experts cannot say for sure, but they do know that protein buffers plaque acid. The casein (milk protein) found in dairy products actually reduces plaque's ability to stick to teeth. To make the most of balanced meals, serve children cookies or ice cream right after meals, rather than between them.

Water Worries

Bottled water, and water filtered at home, may not be the best choice for curbing cavities because of low fluoride levels. A majority of the bottled water brands do not contain enough fluoride to combat cavity formation, according to the American Dental Association.

Using bottled water that lacks fluoride to make infant formula is particularly problematic, since formula is the sole or predominant food source in infants under the age of six months and a major source of calories for months thereafter. In older children, when bottled water with inadequate fluoride is consumed more often than fully fluoridated water, it doesn't provide enough protection for teeth. Cooking foods such as pasta and rice in fluoridated water can increase their fluoride content several-fold, however. Find out whether the water your baby or child drinks at day care contains fluoride, and contact the bottler of your brand of water to get the current fluoride concentration. Check back with them every six months to a year, since levels may fluctuate.

Home water filtration systems may be equally harmful to teeth, since they can filter out a good deal of fluoride that's been added to a community water supply. Reverse osmosis and distillation units remove significant amounts of fluoride, although the type, quality, and age of the filters figures into the amount of fluoride that's actually removed. Families who want to use a home filtration system should have their filtered water tested for fluoride, and then speak to their dentist or pediatrician about the possibility of supplemental fluoride for their child.

DIABETES

Diabetes is nearly always a genetic disorder that prevents the body from producing or properly using insulin. Insulin is the hormone that promotes the cells' consumption of glucose from the blood. Glucose is the fuel for all of your body's cells. The energy in the foods your child eats is converted to glucose.

When glucose cannot make its way into the cells, blood glucose levels soar and stay dangerously high. Chronically elevated glucose concentrations in the blood irreversibly damage blood vessels in many parts of the body, which may lead to the complications of diabetes, including vision loss and blindness; heart disease; nerve damage; kidney disease; and, in the long run, foot and leg amputations.

Diabetes comes in two major forms: type 1 (formerly known as insulin-dependent diabetes) and type 2 (once called non-insulin dependent diabetes). A much less prevalent type, gestational diabetes, affects an estimated 4 percent of pregnant women. It typically disappears after giving birth but may lead to diabetes later in life. Diabetes may also be a result of illness, such as cancer, that affects the pancreas. The pancreas is the organ that produces insulin.

In type 1 diabetes, the body kills off its own insulin-producing cells located in the pancreas, making daily insulin shots a must. Type 1 is much less common than type 2 but is the predominant form of diabetes in children and young adults. Out of the nearly 16 million people with diabetes, about 15 million of them have the type 2 variety. People with type 2 diabetes are poor producers of insulin. In addition, they are usually *insulin resistant,* so even if they make enough insulin, their cells can't use it properly.

Determining Diabetes

Some of the signs of diabetes, including irritability and fatigue, can throw parents, who may mistake them for lack of sleep or stress. In children, diabetes red flags may even mimic the flu. Other symptoms are more dramatic and easier to spot in a child. Talk to your doctor if your child has any of the following symptoms:

- Excessive urination, including chronic bedwetting
- Unquenchable thirst
- Out-of-control hunger despite weight loss and a failure to grow properly
- Dehydration, with dry lips, sunken eyes, and a lack of tears when crying

Historically, type 2 diabetes has been confined to adulthood. But a disturbing trend is emerging among American youth: More than ever, children are developing type 2 diabetes. This phenomenon is alarming on many fronts. Most of the new type 2 cases occur in youngsters 10 or older, but children as young as 4 have the disorder, too. About 85 percent of the children diagnosed with type 2 diabetes are overweight and have a family history of diabetes. According to the American Diabetes Association, children with type 2 diabetes have many more years during which they can develop the harmful side effects of chronically elevated blood glucose levels. Children with type 2 diabetes are at risk for the same complications as anyone with diabetes, including children with the type 1 variety.

Derailing Diabetes: Strategies to Head It Off

You cannot alter your family history of diabetes. Does that mean you can't do anything to head off the condition? That depends. Diabetes is not always completely under your control. For example, some people with type 2 diabetes are neither overweight nor inactive; others with type 1 have no known family history of the condition. Still others have diabetes in their genes but don't get the disease, despite unhealthy habits. Nevertheless, there is a multitude of healthy tactics than can thwart diabetes in your child even as she matures.

Breastfeed your baby. Children with a sibling or parent with diabetes are considered most vulnerable. You probably can't put off type 1 diabetes, given its nearly overwhelming genetic component. Type 1 diabetes is an autoimmune disease, meaning that the body turns against itself for unknown reasons, destroying the cells of the pancreas that produce insulin. However, breastfeeding provides a ray of hope, in part because it boosts immunity. Some researchers suspect a connection between cow's-milk protein in any form (including infant formula) and increased diabetes risk in susceptible children. It seems that giving cow's-milk protein to infants genetically prone to diabetes causes the body to destroy the specific cells in the pancreas responsible for insulin production. This theory has yet to be borne out in controlled scientific studies, however. Even without solid proof of the connection between consuming infant formula and regular milk and diabetes risk, the AAP recommends avoiding cow's milk and products containing cow's-milk protein until after a susceptible child's first birthday.

Weight control. Most of the children with type 2 diabetes are obese. Weight control can help thwart type 2 diabetes in childhood and in adulthood. Excess fat promotes the insulin resistance that results in elevated blood glucose levels. Insulin resistance is typically reversed with weight loss.

Move it. Exercise spurs muscles to take up more glucose from the bloodstream, effectively lowering elevated levels to a more normal range. The evidence for exercise as a way to reduce diabetes risk is compelling. Walking just thirty minutes a day greatly reduces the risk of developing type 2 diabetes in adults and may benefit kids, too.

OSTEOPOROSIS

Chances are good that you've been affected by osteoporosis in one way or another. Perhaps a parent, grandparent, or aunt has broken a hip. Maybe you've heard of an older person who has easily fractured a bone. Or you could have the beginnings of osteoporosis yourself. That's to be expected, since osteoporosis affects nearly 28 million Americans.

Half of all American women will break a bone during their lifetime because of osteoporosis, most likely a hip or a bone in the spine. In fact, a female's risk for hip fracture is equal to her combined risk for breast, uterine, and ovarian cancer, according to the National Osteoporosis Foundation.

Most of the victims are older females. Yet, osteoporosis is by no means a disease of "old age." Quite the opposite: The process leading to osteoporosis begins in the preadolescent years and is often the sum of a lifetime of poor health habits and other factors.

The National Institutes of Health says osteoporosis must begin in childhood. While age-related bone loss figures into osteoporosis risk, youngsters who fail to build the necessary bone mass as children and teenagers are prone to osteoporosis later in life.

Bone Up

Bones suffer from an image problem. They appear hard and static from the outside. But their solid stature belies what goes on inside. Underneath their tough exterior, bones bustle with activity, undergoing a perpetual makeover called remodeling. As bone tissue donates and receives nutrients such as calcium, it is constantly being broken down and built up again. You may not be getting any taller as an adult, but that doesn't mean you should ignore your bones. An unhealthy lifestyle hurts bones, leading to osteoporosis, a crippling disease that causes bones to deteriorate.

Better Bones Start Here

You can't protect your child from getting older, nor can you shield her from a family history of osteoporosis—two factors contributing to the condition. You can do plenty to encourage a lifestyle to build and maintain strong bones in your youngster, however.

Guiding girls toward a healthy lifestyle is paramount for preventing osteoporosis decades later. Women, particularly smaller, thinner-boned females, have less bone tissue than men and lose bone more rapidly, increasing the chances for osteoporosis. In addition, menopause at any age and for any reason sharply decreases levels of the bone-protecting hormone estrogen, causing bone loss to accelerate. Caucasian and Asian women are at particular risk, although African American and Hispanic American women are at significant risk, too.

How Much Calcium and Vitamin D for You and Your Family?

Age determines calcium and vitamin D needs. Check the chart below for how much calcium each family member requires.

Age (years)	Recommended Calcium Daily Intake (milligrams)	Recommended Vitamin D Daily Intake (International Units)
1–3	500	200
4–8	800	200
9–13	1,300	200
14–18	1,300	200
19–30	1,000	200
31–50	1,000	200
51–70	1,200	400
71 plus	1,200	600
Pregnant, 18 or under	1,300	200
Pregnant, 18 plus	1,000	200
Lactating 18 or under	1,300	200
Lactating, 18 plus	1,000	200

Here's how to help your child build stronger bones for life.

Discourage smoking. Cigarette smoking weakens bones. Be a role model for your child. Don't smoke.

Review medications with your pediatrician. Certain medications taken on a regular basis can cause calcium loss. Steroids used to manage asthma or rheumatoid arthritis in kids leach calcium from bones. Check all medications with your child's doctor. Your youngster may need more calcium.

Promote play. Playing builds bone tissue. Encourage your kids to play outside. Just a few minutes of strong summer sunshine most days of the week will initiate the vitamin D production that fosters bone strength, even when they are wearing sunscreen.

Encourage a healthy weight. Help your child achieve and maintain a healthy weight for life. Being too thin as a result of eating inadequate calories and protein can actually suppress estrogen levels in adolescent girls. Estrogen is a hormone that helps foster strong bones.

Serve healthy foods. See "Eat Your Way to Stronger Bones."

Eat Your Way to Stronger Bones

Truth is, you can't control most of the risk factors for osteoporosis, but you can manage many of them, including diet.

Bones and teeth pack nearly all the calcium the body contains. Most bone calcium is deposited there during childhood and early adulthood, which makes this time of life truly critical for preventing bone disease later on. Your heart and muscles require some calcium to function, so calcium floats around in the bloodstream, too. The body must maintain that level at all times to keep running in top form.

Bones are the body's bank for calcium. When levels of calcium are adequate in the blood, calcium is deposited in bones, partly as a reserve for when the levels of calcium drop in the bloodstream. When blood calcium levels get too low, the body makes calcium withdrawals from bones. Vitamin D helps facilitate these ongoing deposits and withdrawals.

A child's calcium intake tends to fall off with age. Teenage girls have notoriously deficient calcium intakes. Only 10 percent of girls ages nine to seventeen take in the calcium they need to build bones that will last; only 25 percent of boys get enough calcium. Set the stage for your youngster's teenage years by helping her or him get enough calcium now.

Is Soy the Solution?

In their natural state, soy beverages contain traces of calcium and vitamin D. Fortified soy beverages are better choices but may not provide as much calcium as you think. A study published in the *American Journal of Clinical Nutrition* has found that the calcium found naturally in milk is more efficiently absorbed by the body than the calcium added to soy drinks. That doesn't mean that you cannot obtain calcium from soy beverages, but it does mean that you should choose drinks that state they provide more than 30 percent of the DV for calcium (the amount found in cow's milk) per eight ounces. Look for soy and milk beverages that contain added vitamin D.

Vitamin D is often passed over as a contributor to bone strength. Without vitamin D, calcium wouldn't be worth much to your child's bones. That's because vitamin D regulates blood calcium levels, encourages the incorporation of calcium into bones, and prevents faulty bone development and bone disease, including osteoporosis.

The body makes vitamin D, and you also get some through food. Sunlight sparks vitamin D production, which begins in skin and ends in the liver and kidneys. Healthy people who are exposed to ten to fifteen minutes of sun most summer days typically make enough vitamin D, storing excess in their livers to be used as needed. People living in colder climates have less vitamin D on board because they make less due to lack of adequate sunlight.

In their natural state, most foods are actually poor vitamin D sources. Nearly all the milk produced in the United States is fortified with vitamin D, however.

Vitamin C is best known for its role in boosting immunity, namely in fighting off colds. So it probably comes as a surprise that vitamin C bolsters bone strength, too. How? Vitamin C plays a role in the production of collagen. Collagen is found in all types of connective tissue and in bones.

Vitamin K, found in green leafy vegetables such as lettuce, broccoli, and Brussels sprouts, jump-starts the production of osteocalcin, a bone protein vital to skeletal strength.

OVERWEIGHT AND OBESITY

Kids are getting fatter at younger ages in this country. It's really no wonder when you consider that a third of American adults are overweight. Studies show that when parents are overweight, so, too, are their children. Likewise, sedentary parents tend to have children who are less physically active than parents who lead a more active lifestyle.

From a health perspective, it's one thing to gain ten pounds in your thirties or forties, but quite another to carry around extra fat starting at four or five years old, which is happening at an unprecedented rate in American children. More than 10 percent of preschoolers ages four to five weigh more than they should as compared to less than 6 percent nearly thirty years ago. The trend is alarming, since it's much more difficult to reverse obesity in young children than it is to prevent it. When kids gain excess fat early in life, it becomes harder for them to overcome obesity. Being overweight during adolescence translates into increased risk for heart disease, high blood pressure, atherosclerosis, colon cancer, gout, and arthritis during adulthood. To add insult to injury, children who carry their weight around their midsections (apple shaped) are more likely than their pear-shaped counterparts to have higher blood triglyceride (fat) levels and lower HDL-cholesterol values; higher blood pressure; and a larger left ventricle, the region of the heart that enlarges in order to work harder to pump blood in overweight individuals.

Is Your Child Overweight?

It takes more than stepping on the scale to determine whether your child weighs too much. The Body Mass Index (BMI) assesses a person's body weight relative to height and is useful for most family members. For all its simplicity—it takes little more than a reliable scale and a calculator—BMI is remarkably telling.

For adults, a BMI between 25 and 29.9 means you're overweight; you're obese if you come out with a BMI of 30 or above. Scientific studies say as BMI levels rise, so, too, does blood pressure and total cholesterol levels in many adults. While BMI is a fairly reliable low-tech test for most people, it has a pitfall. Highly muscular adolescents and adults may appear overweight according to the BMI standards, even though they are not overly fat. That's because muscle weighs more than fat.

In children ages two and older, BMI is a good indicator of body fat, but the parameters for assessing overweight and obesity are different for youngsters. For kids, a BMI that exceeds the 85th percentile on pediatric growth charts indicates obesity may be in the offing.

Here's how to figure BMI.

1. Weigh your child naked.
2. Confirm his height in inches.
3. Multiply his weight in pounds by 705.
4. Divide the result in #3 by his height in inches.
5. Divide the result in #4 by his height in inches again. That's his BMI.

What causes kids to become overweight? In most children, it's probably a mixture of genetic tendency and environment. Unlike adults, kids can make new fat cells, and their fat cells have the capacity to increase in size to accommodate extra calories not expended through physical activity. Once you make fat cells, you never get rid of them, but they do shrink with weight loss. Chromosomal defects and other medical conditions result in obesity, but they are rare.

When is weight a concern? Obesity at age three and older is much more connected to adult obesity than having an overweight infant. In fact, chubby kids under age three who do not have one or more obese parents are at low risk for obesity later in life according to a study in the *New England Journal of Medicine*. You may have cause for concern when your child's weight at any age makes it difficult for her to catch her breath when playing or if it in any way interferes with her ability to socialize with her peers.

Avoiding Obesity: Strategies for Success

Work closely with your pediatrician. If your child appears overweight, have your doctor evaluate her BMI and use it along with pediatric growth charts to determine if she is indeed too heavy. Your child is considered at risk when her BMI exceeds the 85th percentile; and is overweight if she falls above the 95th percentile. According to the AAP, doctors should check the levels of thyroid hormones in obese infants. The thyroid is an organ that helps regulate body weight; when it's sluggish, weight gain can easily occur. Overweight children and their families should seek counsel from a registered dietitian.

Obese Kids Have . . .

- A higher risk for high blood pressure, elevated blood cholesterol and LDL-cholesterol, and reduced HDL-cholesterol
- A harder time breathing
- A larger left chamber of the heart, which boosts heart disease risk
- More upper respiratory infections
- Reduced immunity
- Earlier puberty and irregular periods in girls
- Increased levels of insulin in the blood
- Increased psychological stress, including low self-esteem during adolescence, and increased risk for risky behaviors such as smoking cigarettes and consuming alcohol
- More orthopedic problems

Turn it off. Studies show a strong connection between television watching and childhood obesity. That makes sense, since kids don't burn nearly as many calories parked in front of a TV set—or computer, for that matter—as they do swinging from a jungle gym or playing tag. With the advent of clickers, kids don't even have to get up off the couch to change the channel. The AAP advises limiting television and computer time to no more than two hours a day for children over the age of two. What they're viewing matters, too. Commercial television is rife with advertisements for foods packed with sugar and fat and largely devoid of nutrients. If kids must watch TV, make it a limited amount of Public Broadcasting System programming to minimize negative food messages.

Children who eat high-fat snacks while watching television add insult to injury. That's because they are less likely to pay attention to feelings of fullness and will probably end up consuming excess calories.

Limit high-calorie foods. Kids should curb their consumption of highly refined foods such as cookies, cakes, ice cream, sugary drinks, and snack chips. These choices are packed with calories, so small amounts make for large energy intakes. And they taste so good that it's easy to eat too much. But beware of reduced-fat foods. They may be just as high or even higher in calories than their counterparts because manufacturers add sugar to compensate for missing fat.

Low-Calorie Lowdown

Lower calorie foods dominate the dairy case, clutter the cookie and cracker aisle, and overrun condiment shelves. They're everywhere, but do low-calorie foods aid in weight loss? You would think artificially sweetened beverages, low-fat crackers and snack chips, and fat-free frozen desserts would have slimmed us down by now. Truth is, Americans are heavier than ever, despite the burgeoning reduced-calorie food industry.

What's going on? We're eating more than we need. Just because a food contains fewer calories doesn't mean we can eat larger portions without negative consequences, including weight gain.

The upside of low-calorie foods is that when they are used judiciously, they do foster weight control. Consider the calorie-cutting ability of skim and 1% low-fat milk; fat-free yogurt; reduced-calorie breads; and lower fat mayonnaise, salad dressing, and margarine. As long as you don't overdo it, low-calorie foods are worth the investment for adults, but they are not always appropriate for children.

Attack the snacks. One recent study suggests that snacking in two- to eighteen-year-olds is partially responsible for increasing calorie intakes. Most children need snacks, but between-meal noshing tends to be a high-calorie affair that can easily lead to weight gain. Even fifty unnecessary calories a day can result in enough calories eaten over a year's time to equal more than five pounds of body fat. The remedy? Schedule healthy meals and snacks as much as possible. Don't allow a child to drink milk or juice at will all day long. Keep foods out of reach, and let kids know that they should ask you first before pulling up a chair to the counter to get at the cookie jar.

Take the lead. Kids with one or more overweight parents are more likely to become obese as children and stay that way. Parents are busy, but you must do what you can to foster a healthy weight in your child. Shopping for and preparing reduced-calorie meals that are tasty and nutritious benefit the entire family, and set the tone for how your child should eat.

Avoid focusing on body weight. There is a social stigma attached to being overweight. Indicating your concern about your youngster's body weight can backfire, sending him to seek comfort in food even when his weight is acceptable. What's more, being overweight can isolate a child from his peers, so the less you say about the matter, the better.

Don't eliminate, moderate. All foods fit into a healthy diet for weight control, but in limited amounts. How often you allow your child to eat certain foods should depend on their nutritional merit.

In My Experience
It's a Family Affair

Want your children to eat well and control their weight? Change your own dietary habits for the better first. The studies paint a grim picture when it comes to weight control success: Even when overweight children lose weight, 80 to 90 percent of them gain it back. Yet, the youngsters that I have seen for weight control do the best when the entire family is geared toward eating a more healthy diet. As a parent or other loving caregiver, your actions speak louder than words. Not surprisingly, researchers writing in the *International Journal of Eating Disorders* found that 77 percent of the young children they spoke with said their parents and relatives were their primary source of weight control information. Yet, you can preach the benefits of carrots over snack chips to your children, but the advice won't stick with them unless you eat the way you want them to. Researchers at Boston University School of Medicine have found that children ages three to five of parents who either eat impulsively or who consciously restrict food became heavier than children of parents who did neither. Either way, it seems that the parents in the study failed to listen to their own internal hunger or fullness cues. Kids pick up on that, and will mimic the behavior.

Love your body. Bodies come in all shapes and sizes. Your child should be encouraged to love hers, but that can't happen unless you stop talking about your own physical faults, or those of your spouse. Kids are very much aware of how others perceive them, and they are sensitive to societal cues about body image as well. A study in the *International Journal of Eating Disorders* has found that children as young as eight are worried about the shape of their bodies, which researchers say makes them vulnerable to eating disorders and depression.

Move It

A decline in physical activity and regular exercise may be largely to blame for the fattening of American children, which in turn results in greater risk of a host of health problems, least of which is heart disease and diabetes. Data from consumption studies show that calorie intakes among most age groups have not increased, yet obesity is on the rise. That means kids are not moving around enough.

According to the Dietary Guidelines for Americans, children should aim for at least sixty minutes of physical activity a day. But a survey conducted for the International Life Sciences Institute has found that fewer than one in four children get twenty minutes of vigorous daily physical activity every day. That means they are missing out on the benefits of exercise.

Exercise:

- Fosters physical fitness, including endurance and muscular strength
- Builds strong bones and joints
- Burns calories
- Keeps blood pressure in check
- Promotes well-being
- Reduces stress and feelings of depression and anxiety

Parents of sedentary children must take the lead to get their kids to exercise regularly. Take your children to the playground as often as possible, and take walks with them when you can. Any activity is good for kids, including jumping rope, playing tag, riding a bike or a tricycle, climbing on a jungle gym, rollerblading, dancing, tumbling, walking, hiking, skiing, skating, martial arts, and sledding.

Linger at mealtimes. Encourage children to eat slowly by engaging them in conversation. Slowing down will better preserve a child's keen ability to regulate his food intake. When your youngster tells you that he is full but his meal is half-done, listen to what he's saying and don't make him finish. Let your child respond to his own physical cues for hunger and fullness.

Breastfeed your baby. Research out of Germany suggests that five- and six-year-olds who were nursed the longest as babies before beginning formula or food were far less likely to be overweight.

Enlist the help of family members and day care providers. Grandparents, aunts and uncles, babysitters, and any other adult that spends a lot of time with your child must know about any weight concerns you have. But be discreet, and be reasonable. Do not discuss your efforts to control your youngster's weight in her presence.

Diets don't work. Don't restrict your child's food without first checking with your doctor or dietitian. Children under the age of six have elevated nutrient needs. Cutting back on food without professional guidance can jeopardize your child's development.

Don't use food as a bribe or a remedy. Promising your son candy if he is good while you shop at the mall or handing him a lollipop every time he scrapes his knee distorts his inborn ability to regulate food intake based on hunger. Reward your child by spending time with him instead of giving him food.

Chapter 14

Your Child's Food Away from Home

Keep 'em busy
and feed them first.

—Cindy, mother of two boys,
on how to handle kids in restaurants

FAMILY FARE: DINING OUT WITH YOUNGSTERS

When our two oldest were very young, we would dine out nearly every Saturday night. I found Hayley, two, and Hannah, one, fairly easy to handle in restaurants, perhaps because we had begun taking them out as newborns. As long as we met their needs first, the girls were near-perfect dinner companions (and still are). Taking them along meant Tom and I got a chance to try out some local, moderately priced restaurants without paying a babysitter. Even with three kids in tow, our family eats away from home at least once a week, even if it means fast food at the mall. Hayley, Hannah, and Emma love to go out for breakfast, lunch, dinner, and snacks (did someone say donuts?), and overall, unless someone is having a bad day, the girls are great companions. They are so well behaved and easy to manage in public that my husband or I can take all three out by ourselves without incident.

It may sound like I'm bragging, and I probably am to some degree. I'm proud that they behave well in restaurants and even enjoy going out. Perhaps we are lucky, but I think that their behavior is based on some hard work on our part. Tom and I have never avoided taking our children with us when dining out. Eating in restaurants is part of our fast-paced lifestyle, and we also see it as a way to expose the children to different types of cuisine.

The ease of takeout fare and restaurant dining is what attracts busy families, especially when both parents work. According to the National Restaurant Association, Americans over the age of eight eat away from the home more than four times a week, or nearly two hundred times a year. It's probably safe to say that many individuals and families don't dine out as much as statistics suggest, however. In fact, a survey by *Restaurants and Institutions* found that couples without children dine out about 30 percent more often than couples with kids. For some people, dining out is a rare pleasure to be savored and enjoyed. If this description fits you, you'll be tempted to leave your child at home when you crave a quiet meal and good conversation. But don't do it too often. Your son could become uncomfortable in restaurant settings, so that when you dine out with him, the meal is chaotic.

Strategies for Successful Dining with Kids

Tom and I have ways of handling the children in a restaurant setting that work best for us. We are not above using as many tricks and techniques as possible to ensure a more pleasant meal. The more prepared you are, the better. Here are tried-and-true strategies, some more obvious than others.

Choose a conducive restaurant with attentive wait staff. Eating establishments that cater to kids rank high on our list. Choose restaurants that offer good service and pleasant decor to get the most from your dining experience. We have several favorites that we know are accepting of children. We especially favor places that offer coloring materials and have high chairs and booster seats that are in good condition.

Request an out-of-the-way table or booth. When the hostess sees us coming, I imagine she's thinking about where to put us so that we won't disrupt the other diners, which is usually in a section designated for families. That's fine by me, as long as I can get good service. If you prefer a booth in a more central location, let the wait staff or hostess know your wishes.

Lower your expectations. Your significant other may be present and there may even be a candle on the table. Don't get any ideas. This is no romantic dinner. Save that type of dining for another time and focus on the children.

Go early. For the most part, we try to make it to a restaurant by 6:00 P.M., especially on weekend nights. Places are much less crowded, so it's easier to get the seating we need, the service is better, and the kids tend to be less cranky at that time of day.

Relax. You don't have to cook or clean up. What could be better? (Kids who behaved perfectly, maybe?)

Keep kids occupied. As my friend Cindy suggests, bring crayons and coloring books or paper, books, or small (noiseless, please) toys to keep kids from climbing the wall while waiting for their food to arrive.

Don't make them wait. Young children do not operate on your schedule. They can become very hungry while waiting for their meal. A hungry child can be whiny and unruly, so bring along some low-fat snacks such as carrot sticks, pretzels, or crackers to take the edge off hunger. Offer kids a roll or some snack chips while they wait. We order the kids' meals well before we place our order, and then get them a bowl of ice cream to eat while we're eating our meal. Since Tom and I rarely order dessert, this works out great as far as timing because everyone is done at about the same time.

Focus on the familiar, but encourage new foods, too. Children crave routine, and it's no different when they dine out. You may look forward to trying a new cuisine, but they may have other things in mind. As I mentioned, Hayley and Hannah typically request fried chicken nuggets and French fries or rice if they're not eating pizza, another favorite. Recently, we took them to their first-ever Thai restaurant, where the only offering close to chicken nuggets was chicken sate with peanut sauce. Being creatures of habit, I thought they would reject it. Turns out, they loved the chicken sate. They even went for our sticky rice, which had a different feel and taste than the boiled white rice we had ordered for them. At that same Thai meal, Hannah ate a healthy serving of noodles from our pad thai dish, also something new for her.

Dining, Discounted

Dining out with a family can tax your budget, but there are ways to cut costs. Here's how.

- *Be an early bird.* Eating between 4:00 and 6:00 P.M. is good for hungry kids and can save you a bundle in restaurants offering Early Bird Specials.
- *Go out to breakfast.* Lunch and dinner tend to be costlier than breakfast. Plus, kids have more energy in the morning and tend to be less cranky.
- *Cash in on two-for-one offers.* Local newspapers contain coupons that allow you and a companion to purchase two entrees for the price of one.
- *Don't sit down.* Takeout foods cost much less than when you sit down to eat. Grab the food and go home. It will save you a bundle on beverages and a tip.
- *Buffets.* All-you-can eat extravaganzas are attractive, and they may actually be worth it for a family. Check out the children's price before digging in.
- *Split an entree with your significant other.* You'll save money and calories. Ask for half-portions of regular entrees.

Include fruit or vegetables. You may not be able to get them to eat a salad or a side order of broccoli, but that doesn't mean dining out must be devoid of produce. Hayley adores the pineapple presented at the end of a Chinese meal and eats nearly the whole portion when it arrives. As long as fruit is on the menu in some form, you don't have to wait until the end of the meal to ask for it. Include a fruit cup with your child's meal, or order juice instead of soda. Baked potatoes instead of French fries are also a more nutritious option, even when covered in sour cream.

ON THE MENU

The kids may order the same things every time they go out to eat, but not you. You're looking for something delicious and nutritious. Make sure you pass over high-fat options including onion soup, Caesar salad, taco salad, mashed potatoes, fried chicken strips or nuggets, coleslaw, Cobb salad, broccoli-and-cheese-stuffed potatoes, and scones.

Avoid the pitfalls of a variety of cuisines with these helpful hints.

Flagging Fat

Restaurant food isn't always what it seems. Broiled fish sounds like it's designed for people watching their waistlines, but it can be smothered in butter or margarine when it arrives at your table. The pasta primavera that sounds so healthy could come tossed in a cheese sauce. It pays to learn the lingo and to ask questions about how your food is prepared. These menu terms translate into high-fat fare:

- Basted
- Batter dipped
- Buttery
- Creamy
- Crispy
- Deep fried
- Grande
- Pan fried
- Parmesan
- Supreme

Chinese

Think Chinese food is light? Not always. Many popular dishes are full of hidden fat.

Problems
- Copious quantities of oil in stir-fries and in deep fat frying
- High-fat meats such as spare ribs and fried chicken or shrimp

Solutions
- Share the calories. Split entrees.
- Use chopsticks so you'll eat slowly. Teach your kids how to use them, too.
- Ask your server to have the chef prepare your food with a minimum of oil.
- Order steamed rice instead of fried rice and noodle dishes.
- Try tofu dishes, but not if the tofu is deep-fried.
- Go for entrees packing chicken, bean curd (tofu), or seafood and an abundance of vegetables.

Italian
Problems
- Large portions
- Lots of cheese
- Liberal use of olive oil

Solutions
- Split entrees.
- Order plainer items such as pasta with marinara sauce, grilled fish, or roasted or grilled chicken, or lighter veal dishes such as veal marsala.
- Order plenty of fresh vegetables.
- Take it easy on the olive oil.
- Go for cappuccino over cannoli or tiramisu for dessert.

Fast Food
Fast food is attractive to families. It's cheap and it's fast, but it's hardly healthy, as a rule.

Problems
- Supersize meals are tempting because you get more for your money.
- Fish and chicken sandwiches are nearly always fried, and so are chicken nuggets or chicken strips.
- Overall, fast food fare packs excessive amounts of calories, fat, and sodium.

Solutions
- Seek out fast food joints with healthier offerings, including chili, baked potatoes, and salads.
- Downsize your meal. Think of the size of fries you want, then go one size lower. Ditto for drinks, unless it's milk or juice.
- Purchase a supersize meal and have children share it.
- Add a salad with low-calorie dressing.

Mexican
Take a few of the chips awaiting you at the table and ask to have the rest removed. That way, no one will be too full for dinner.

Problems
- Packed with cheese and high-fat guacamole
- Much of the food is high-fat because it is fried
- Few fresh vegetables

Solutions

- Order bean soup or chili and a dinner salad.
- Skip condiments such as sour cream, and try to pull off most of the cheese.
- Stick with bean and chicken enchiladas or burritos, fajitas, and tacos.
- Forgo dessert unless you plan to split it at least four ways.

Yeah, But Is It Really Good for You?

Meals touted as healthy that are served on airplanes, in delis, or in a fine restaurant must adhere to the same rules as food you buy in a store. By law, restaurants and airlines must substantiate their health claims about commercially prepared food in much the same way that food companies must back up the language on their food labels, according to the FDA. Consumers can demand the information on the spot, but eating establishments and airlines are not responsible for posting nutrition information for the public.

Pizza

Friday nights are pizza night at our house. The kids really look forward to it, even Emma, who at eighteen months knows what pizza is and thoroughly enjoys it. Lucky for us, our kids favor cheese pizza, so it's easy to curb the calories contained in the deep-dish, stuffed-crust varieties and pizzas laden with meat. I always serve the children fruit or vegetables along with the pizza, and I encourage them to drink milk or juice with the meal. Tom and I eat a large green salad with low-fat dressing to avoid overdoing it on the pizza.

Problems

- Fatty toppings and crusts
- Large portions

Solutions

- Order thin-crust pizzas topped with vegetables instead of fatty meats.
- Have fruit or vegetables with your meal to curb pizza consumption.

Thai

Like Chinese fare, Thai food is served family style, making it perfect for sharing, which can conserve calories.

Problems

- Curry. It's made with coconut milk, which is very high in total and

saturated fat.
- Lard, also laden with saturated fat, is often used to prepare traditional Thai foods.
- Peanut sauce and chopped peanuts abound in Thai cuisine, which is a threat to children and adults who are allergic.

Solutions
- Share your entree with other family members.
- Choose chicken, seafood, and bean curd dishes that aren't smothered in curry or peanut sauce.
- Avoid Thai iced coffee and Thai iced tea as they contain cream and sugar.

Takeout Trends

It's 4:00 P.M. Do you have a clue what to serve for dinner? If you're like most American adults, the answer is no. According to a survey conducted by *Restaurants and Institutions*, 71 percent of us don't bother planning the evening meal much before late afternoon, which may account for another finding: Dinner is four times as likely as lunch to be taken out of the restaurant and eaten at home. For busy families, takeout fare and food delivered directly to your door fills in for home-based meal planning and preparation a good deal of the time. When the kids are clamoring for food, you need a speedy dinner. But take care. According to the USDA, on the whole, food made outside of the home contains more fat and saturated fat and less of the beneficial calcium, fiber, and iron that kids need.

DAY CARE CUISINE

With more mothers working full or part time, child care is a fact of life for most families. Nearly 13 million American preschoolers are enrolled in child care programs, according to the National Center for Education Statistics. That means that more than 60 percent of the nation's children ages six and under are supervised during the day by someone other than a parent. As of 1995, a third of the infants and preschoolers enrolled in child care programs participated in center-based care, while 20 percent were cared for in home-based programs. The remainder of the children were supervised by relatives or by a sitter in the child's home.

When parents choose people to care for children in their absence, what do they value? Warmth and caring no doubt come to mind. A safe and nurturing environment is critical, too. Nutrition should be just as important to parents. The quality of the food your child eats while in any child care situation affects his short- and long-term health and well-being. The more time your youngster spends with a sitter, the more important nutrition becomes. Anything less than a high standard for nutrition can set the stage for poor eating habits that your youngster may never outgrow.

In general, parents strongly influence a child's nutritional habits, but other caregivers contribute to a youngster's eating patterns, too. You may not know it, but your child models himself in part after his day care providers. And why not? He may spend upwards of five days a week in other people's care. Chances are, your youngster admires and identifies with the sitter he sees daily or nearly daily.

Ensuring that your child's diet away from home is healthy is crucial for a number of reasons. Surveys show that preschoolers are getting progressively heavier. In fact, the incidence of obesity in these youngsters has doubled in the past twenty years. Young children are not eating adequate fruits, vegetables, or whole grains. Since your child may spend most of her waking hours in the care of others, her diet should be as healthy as possible during that time.

You have a say about what, and how, your child eats while you're at work. Read on.

Child Care Check List

You may be looking for a suitable child care situation, or re-evaluating your current program. In any case, don't forget to ask about the following.

How can parents become involved? What kids eat at day care should be an open book, and any program should welcome your questions about its menus. But it seems that few parents have thought to inquire about what their children eat. Research shows minimal parental involvement with day care diets. It's folly to expect your day care provider to supply your child with the nutrients she needs to grow and develop properly if you don't check on what's being served first.

How often is food offered? The American Dietetic Association suggests children need to consume at least a third of their daily nutrients when in the care of others for four to seven hours. Children in day care for eight hours should expect to satisfy at least half to two-thirds of their daily nutrient requirements.

Unless you provide written instructions to the contrary, your infant should be fed on demand, not according to the sitter's schedule. Be sure to ask your sitter to hold your infant when giving him a baby bottle. Preschoolers should go no longer than three hours before being offered a snack or meal.

How are meals planned? Providers should use the guiding principals of the USDA's Food Guide Pyramid for Young Children (see "Pyramid Power," page 42). Kids should eat at least one source of vitamin C a day, including citrus, tomatoes, kiwis, and strawberries, and be offered good sources of vitamin A, such as carrots and sweet potatoes, at least thrice weekly as part of a well-balanced meal plan.

Does the program participate in the Child and Adult Care Food Program? This is a plus when deciding on day care, according to research. That's because kids tend to eat better when enrolled in programs that participate. Child care programs that enroll in the Child and Adult Care Food Program (CACFP) administered by the USDA have a better track record of supplying children with necessary nutrients. The CACFP reimburses eligible child care programs for the costs of food and foodservice operations, and CACFP participants must receive annual training about child nutrition and the CACFP requirements.

Are foods laden with fat, sugar, and sodium kept to a minimum? There's no need for providers to entice kids to eat by adding fat, sugar, and salt during or after food preparation. Children possess a heightened sense of taste, which is one of the reasons why seasonings are not particularly pleasing to them. Nor should providers offer your youngster too many snacks supplying fat, sugar, and sodium, such as high-fat crackers, cookies, candy, and sugary drinks.

Does your provider post weekly menus? If not, ask if it's possible. That way, you'll be informed about what your child is being served.

What's the procedure for hand washing and other food safety practices? At the very minimum, children should wash their hands with warm soapy water for at least twenty seconds and dry them with a clean dry cloth or paper towel before every meal and snack, after visiting the bathroom, after touching animals, and more frequently when they have a cold. Make sure your day care program provides for this. Likewise, staff should wash their hands after every diaper check or change, after visiting the bathroom, and before and after handling food.

Are food preparation and storage areas neat and clean? Don't forget to check out these areas. Adequate refrigeration is a must. Children bringing food from home should be able to store it in a clean refrigerator that operates at 40°F or below.

Where is the diaper changing area? It should be away from the areas where children eat and play, to minimize the spread of germs.

How much does your child care provider know about nutrition? CACFP participants must receive annual nutrition training, but other day care providers may know less about child nutrition. In fact, research bears that out. In one study, only about half of the caregivers could correctly select the major food sources for certain nutrients (i.e., dairy foods as a source of calcium) or knew the appropriate serving sizes for preschoolers.

Is the environment conducive to eating? The best way to find out is by observing—unannounced. Our sitter Louise, who has been caring for my children for the past five years, allows parents to drop in without notice, a policy that I applaud. The notion that you can walk into your baby-sitter's house, or that you can go unannounced to your day care center, is comforting. What should you look for once you're there? Clean, safe, and cheerful eating areas designed for toddlers and preschoolers. Serving food family style is preferable, but let's face it, it's not always possible when kids are clamoring for their meal and your sitter is scrambling to meet the needs of children of many different ages. As at home, food should never be used as a reward or a punishment at day care; nor should your sitter force a child to eat. Sitters should not allow kids to share food.

Nutrition That Makes the Grade

Surveys suggest that food offered at child care centers and family-based programs may come up short for calories, iron, zinc, and magnesium, which could compromise peak cognitive development in your child. Participating in the USDA's Child and Adult Care Food Program may significantly improve a child's diet, however. According to research published in the *Journal of the American Dietetic Association* comparing an urban-based day care center that participated in the CACFP with one that did not, striking differences were found in the childrens' nutrient intake. Youngsters who brought food from home to eat during the day ate significantly less vitamin A, riboflavin, and calcium compared to those served more wholesome meals and snacks prepared with CACFP guidelines in mind. Researchers also found that the better-nourished children were sick on average four days less during the seven months of the study. Other unrelated research suggests that when a registered dietitian is involved in meal planning, children have access to higher quality foods.

In My Experience
What Sitters Must Know

Never assume a sitter knows what's on your mind in terms of feeding your child, no matter how experienced she is or how well she knows your youngster. Whether you have hired someone to care for your child at home while you work, have arranged for a relative to sit during the day, or take your youngster to a family- or center-based child care program, you must spell out what you want your child to eat. This is especially critical for kids with special needs such as diabetes or celiac disease. My sitters must think me crazy at times, but I always write down what my children should have for meals and snacks before I leave the house.

Make life easier for your sitter by preparing food ahead of time or arranging for them to prepare simple meals such as sandwiches, fruit or vegetables, and milk, which allows for more time spent with your child and less time in the kitchen. For example, when my husband and I go out to dinner without the kids, we order pizza for the kids and the sitter and serve it with fruit. Premixing infant formula and bottling it in the necessary portions helps, too. If you're breastfeeding, do the same to prepare bottles.

I don't own a microwave oven, but if I did, I would tell sitters not to use it to heat baby bottles, and I'd show them how to operate it to avoid burns when heating up prepared foods for older children. On the subject of safety, write down the age-appropriate foods for each child, and warn sitters about the risks of choking in youngsters under the age of four (see page 113 for a list of dangerous foods). Alert all caregivers to your feelings about feeding your child sugary snacks and foods laden with fat and sodium. Make sitters aware of a child's food allergies, what foods to avoid, and the symptoms of an allergic reaction. Although the chances of choking are slim, I feel most comfortable with mature sitters who know how to prevent, and treat, choking in infants and children. Always leave emergency numbers for any sitter.

Chapter 15

Special
Concerns

We respect life,
and we respect animals,
so we don't eat them.
It's really easy for the
kids to be vegetarian
because they are
so attached to animals.
If more people knew
how easy and healthy
it is to forgo meat,
there would be a lot
more vegetarians.

—Carol, *mother of three vegetarian children*

RAISING A VEGETARIAN CHILD

Vegetarianism means different things to different people. The term may be used to (incorrectly) describe a diet that omits red meat but includes chicken and fish, or an eating regimen that excludes all animal products. Vegetarian diets run the gamut. Most American vegetarians are lacto-ovo; they eat dairy products and eggs but eschew meat, poultry, and seafood. Some are ovo-vegetarians who include eggs but no dairy, meat, seafood, or poultry. Other people are vegans, who avoid all animal products, including honey and gelatin.

Parents may prefer vegetarianism for any number of reasons, including moral and religious beliefs, concern for the environment, and disease prevention. No matter how your family eats, you must make sure your child gets the nutrients he needs to thrive. The typical American diet doesn't automatically guarantee that he will, and neither does a vegetarian eating plan.

Hallmarks of Healthy Vegetarianism

People perceive vegetarian diets as healthier than mainstream eating, but is it a preferable eating plan for youngsters? That depends. Several studies show a connection between vegetarian diets and reduced risk for developing certain chronic illnesses, including heart disease, obesity, and certain cancers in adults. The diet and health link remained strong even when researchers factored in the protective effects of regular physical activity and lack of cigarette smoking in the vegetarians. While research on vegetarian youngsters is lacking, it stands to reason that children who eat fewer animal products and more of a plant-based diet beginning early in life would reap similar benefits as they age.

Yet, vegetarian diets are not necessarily healthy ones unless they are well planned. Simply leaving out meat, fish, and fowl doesn't turn a poor mainstream diet into a healthy one, especially when it comes to children. In my practice, I have seen dozens of adult vegetarians complaining of low energy levels and frequent illness, which, after speaking with them, I could attribute in part to a poor diet.

Like everyone else who eats, vegetarians must take care when designing their diets. There are any number of nutrients to consider. For example, when milk is left out of the equation, how will you make up for missing calcium and vitamin D? Iron and zinc are issues for non-meat eaters—what's your plan for getting enough? And are you eating adequate amounts of high-quality protein?

Very young children are in a critical growth period, and missing out on any nutrient such as protein, calcium, or iron could make for irreparable harm. Parents with vegetarian kids should seek the counsel of a registered dietitian to help plan their diet, especially if they are vegan. Here's what you must include to have the healthiest vegetarian child possible.

Calories

Vegetarian or not, youngsters need enough energy to grow properly. This can be a sticking point for vegetarian kids, largely because of the fiber content of their diet. Fiber is the bulky, indigestible portion of plant foods. Kids can easily fill up on low-fat whole grains, fruits, vegetables, and legumes well before they meet their calorie needs. It may seem strange, but your vegetarian child could do with less fiber. Use more refined grains that also contain some fat, such as graham crackers, for snacks instead of raw fruits and vegetables. Don't go overboard trying to restrict fatty foods such as eggs, full-fat dairy products, and nuts and nut butters, since this can exacerbate your child's energy deficit.

Protein

Kids who don't eat enough calories are prone to inadequate protein intake, too. Plant food protein contains all of the essential amino acids (EAAs) your child needs to grow (see the explanation on page 20), but no single plant food such as bread, pasta, rice, or legumes supplies all of the EAAs, which is why vegans must eat a variety of plant foods. For the most part, animal foods provide all of the EAAs youngsters require for growth. Eggs are particularly rich in EAAs; dairy products come very close to eggs' gold standard for protein. Lacto-ovo vegetarian children who consume the correct amounts of eggs and dairy products should have no trouble meeting EAA requirements. Vegans should eat a wide array of plant-based proteins, including soy products, meat analogs, and nuts and nut butters as part of a varied, balanced diet to get their EAAs.

Iron

Iron is paramount to a child's cognitive function and physical development. Its importance is described on page 30. Meat, poultry, and seafood pack particularly high amounts of the type of iron that is well absorbed by your body. (Dairy foods are a poor source of iron, however.) In spite of being a nation of meat eaters, iron deficiency is common in childhood, and there is no evidence to suggest that on the whole, the effects of iron deficiency are any more prevalent among vegetarian children. However, that doesn't mean you shouldn't be vigilant when it comes to your vegetarian child's body-iron stores. Serve baby only iron-fortified formula. Bran flakes, instant oatmeal, Cream of Wheat, spinach, tomato juice, dried apricots, raisins, garbanzo beans, kidney beans, and tofu rank high on the list of kid-friendly plant foods rich in iron. Serve iron-packed fare along with a source of vitamin C such as citrus, tomatoes, kiwi, or strawberries to increase the body's absorption.

Good Taste, Great Protection

As a group, adult vegetarians suffer from less heart disease and high blood pressure and fewer cancers of the lung and colon. Why? Depending on the eating pattern, vegetarian diets contain less total and saturated fat and less cholesterol, contributing in large part to the lower blood cholesterol levels and LDLs in people with meatless diets. Eating less animal protein than the mainstream American diet may promote bone health, too. That's because many of the amino acids in animal protein create an acidic environment in the body that must be buffered by bone calcium, causing your body to deplete its calcium stores. To boot, plant-based eating is typically higher in beneficial folate, as well as the antioxidant vitamins C, E, and carotenoids. Vegetarian diets tend to be rich in protective phytochemicals and filled with fiber.

Calcium and Vitamin D

Vegans avoid dairy products, which means calcium and vitamin D could go missing. Kids need calcium and vitamin D to build bones that will last as long as they do. Vitamin D enhances calcium absorption and deposition into the bone and maintains proper blood levels of calcium needed for muscle contraction and to normalize heartbeat. Cow's milk is the best food source of this dynamic duo; other dairy products lack supplemental vitamin D. Soy and rice "milks" fortified with vitamin D and calcium may be good cow's-milk substitutes (see "Rating the Milks," page 248). Some plant foods such as broccoli, pinto beans, dried figs, soy nuts (not for children under age four), and Brussels sprouts contain calcium that is well absorbed by the body. Juice with added calcium and tofu processed with calcium are suitable calcium sources for vegetarians, but they don't supply vitamin D. In fact, vitamin D is present naturally in very few foods, most notably egg yolks. Certain breakfast cereals supply added vitamin D. My advice: Give your child a children's multivitamin that meets the 100 percent Daily Value (DV) for vitamin D, no matter what his diet. Breastfeeding vegan mothers should also take a multivitamin daily to make sure the vitamin D in their breast milk is up to par.

Vitamin B$_{12}$

Inadequate vitamin B$_{12}$ intake produces anemia and can lead to irreversible nerve damage, which is particularly devastating in developing children. Vitamin B$_{12}$ is unique to living things, which is why vegans are particularly vulnerable to B$_{12}$ shortfalls. Youngsters who eat milk and eggs but no meat, poultry, or seafood may not meet their vitamin B$_{12}$ requirements, either. For supplemental vitamin B$_{12}$, look to fortified foods such as Red Star Vegetarian Support Formula (a nutritional yeast), breakfast cereals with added vitamin B$_{12}$, meat analogs, and soy beverages. However, do not assume meat analogs and soy beverages automatically contain vitamin B$_{12}$, since content varies by product and may change with time. Read the label before purchasing. The breast milk of vegan mothers may lack adequate vitamin B$_{12}$ for baby's neurological development. Breastfeeding mothers and nursing babies would benefit from a mom's daily multivitamin that contains 100 percent of the DV for vitamin B$_{12}$.

Rating the "Milks"

Parents who eschew cow's milk should know that all milk substitutes are not created equal. While the nutrient content of cow's milk is stable across the board, soy and rice beverages differ greatly. Plus, they don't all offer the same nutrients as cow's milk. For example, rice milk contains a mere 1 gram of protein per 8 ounces, compared to the 8 grams in cow's milk. Calcium and vitamin D content vary widely in soy and rice beverages. Look for brands that supply at least 30 percent of the DV for calcium and 25 percent of the DV for vitamin D so that they are comparable to cow's milk for some of the most important nutrients for kids. Nearly all milk processors add vitamin A to cow's milk, but some soy- and rice-beverage makers do not. Purchase brands that offer 10 percent of the DV for vitamin A so that your child doesn't fall short.

Zinc

Children require zinc for a number of bodily functions, the least of which is cell growth and repair and energy production. Zinc is described in detail on page 34. Since animal foods such as beef pack zinc, one of the potential pitfalls of vegetarianism is poor zinc intake. The problem may be two-fold: inadequate zinc intake and zinc absorption that's hampered by other elements of plant foods. For example, vegetarian diets can be high in phytate, a component of plants that curbs the body's zinc absorption. Foods made with refined flour, such as white bread and cornflakes, actually foster zinc absorption. How? Because white flour lacks a husk, the part of wheat that is phytate-rich and hampers zinc uptake by the body. Manufacturers may fortify plant foods with large amounts of zinc to offset any absorption deficiencies. Legumes, peanut butter, wheat germ, fortified grains, yogurt, and cheese make fine zinc choices for vegetarian kids.

Don't Be a Nut: Diets to Avoid

Not all vegetarianism is good for you or your kids. Any diet that eliminates one or more food groups is off limits for any family member. Fruitarianism is a case in point. As the name implies, fruitarians feast on fruit only. The fruit of a plant is considered to be any food that can be taken from the plant without harming it, such as seeds, nuts, grains, and fruit. Fruitarianism is much too restrictive for children and is, in a word, dangerous. Macrobiotics is a bit more mainstream, yet not without its pitfalls. Past studies suggest that this diet, largely based on whole grains, produce, soups, and sometimes fish, made for poor growth in infants and did not supply adequate vitamin B_{12} and calcium. That's probably because it was taken to extremes, given the misunderstandings about the origins of this largely vegetarian diet, which is meant to establish harmony in individuals.

Docosahexanoic Acid (DHA)

Fish and eggs of chickens raised on feed rich in DHA are good sources of this polyunsaturated fat. DHA is critical to brain development and peak cognition in youngsters. It's particularly important during infancy. While the reports are conflicting, vegetarians who eschew eggs and seafood may lack sufficient DHA, according to the American Dietetic Association. Linolenic acid, found in flaxseed, linseed oil, walnuts, walnut oil, and canola oil, can be converted by the body to DHA. The transformation of linolenic acid to DHA is limited, however.

FEEDING A SICK CHILD

Feed a cold, starve a fever. No wait, isn't it starve a cold, feed a fever?

—Karen, *mother of one*

It's neither. Food and fluid are nearly always the best remedies for sick children. Even when your infant or preschooler eats much less, he still reaps nutritional benefits that help speed recovery.

Colds and Ear Infections

Colds are common in babies and toddlers largely because they haven't yet had the chance to build up immunity to dozens of different viruses they encounter. Children in group day care settings frequently have more colds because of their exposure to other children and adults outside of their family unit. A child may catch a cold twelve times in as many months, while adults have about four colds a year, on average.

A cold typically, but not always, precedes an ear infection. Why are kids prone to ear infections? In part it is because of their anatomy. The eustachian tubes that drain fluid and mucus from your child's ears are shorter than adults' tubes. Shorter tubes promote the migration of germs to the inner ear and increase vulnerability to blockages. When fluid cannot drain out of the eustachian tubes and down the back of the throat, a buildup of bacteria-breeding fluid ensues and ear infection results.

For colds and ear infections, fluids are a must. They help clear mucus and thin secretions. Commercially prepared frozen pops or homemade juice pops or juice cubes help kids get the fluids they need. Warm soups such as chicken are soothing foods that help loosen nasal mucus, providing nourishment and temporary relief. There's no need to restrict dairy products during colds and ear infections, although some pediatricians recommend limiting milk products as a way of reducing mucus.

The Facts on Fever

Your child has a temperature, but don't panic yet. As long as it doesn't go too high (always ask your pediatrician about this), fever indicates the immune system is hard at work fending off germs. Increased body temperature raises your child's fluid and calorie needs. A feverish body needs nourishment to continue doing battle. The irony is that feverish children typically have limited appetites. While you're waiting for her temperature to return to normal, encourage water and diluted fruit juice consumption. Don't skimp on added fat such as butter, margarine, or peanut butter for toddlers and preschoolers—these boost calorie intake without increasing the amount of food your child eats.

Diarrhea

When a child has diarrhea, the lining of his intestinal tract is inflamed. That throws out of whack the normal water balance needed to form firm stools, and he ends up with watery bowel movements. Diarrhea may be caused by a number of factors, but it's typically the result of a virus. The rotavirus is to blame for most bouts of acute diarrhea in kids that typically last five to eight days.

Don't Delay

Experts from the National Institute of Diabetes and Digestive and Kidney Diseases recommend contacting your doctor if any of the following appear in your child:

- Stools containing blood or pus
- Black stools
- Temperature of 101.4°F or above (babies three months and younger: rectal temperature of 100.4°F)
- No improvement within twenty-four hours
- Signs of dehydration:
  - Thirst
  - Less frequent urination
  - Dry skin
  - Fatigue
  - Light-headedness
  - Dry mouth and tongue
  - No tears when crying
  - No wet diapers for three hours or more
  - Sunken abdomen, eyes, or cheeks
  - High fever
  - Listlessness or irritability
  - Skin that does not flatten when pinched and released

While uncomfortable, most cases of diarrhea are not usually harmful. Yet, diarrhea can be serious. Chronic diarrhea in children six months and under is a red flag and should be reported to your doctor. Infants with this condition can easily become malnourished and fail to grow properly.

Prolonged, profuse diarrhea results in life-threatening dehydration. In fact, dodging dehydration is the number one concern in childhood diarrhea. Diarrhea causes a net loss of fluid and the electrolytes sodium, potassium, and chloride from your child's body. Electrolytes regulate nerve impulses, muscle contraction, and fluid balance, so a shortfall spells trouble. Don't hesitate to call your doctor's office for advice, especially if your infant has diarrhea.

Food As Medicine

Getting your child back to normal while dealing with diarrhea means feeding him as soon as possible. Never withhold food because you want to "rest" your child's bowel. Deficient diets can prolong diarrhea, since the gut needs nutrients to heal. Without good nutrition, the lining of the intestine cannot repair itself to the point of improving nutrient absorption, and your child's overall health may suffer as a result.

A regular diet of tolerable foods, including bananas, rice, applesauce, toast (made from low-fiber bread), eggs, and plain pasta are among those foods that speed recovery. Limit sugary foods and high-fiber choices. Full-strength juices, most sports drinks, and soda actually exacerbate diarrhea because the body pulls water into the intestine from the surrounding tissues to dilute the sugar in these drinks. Juices with high levels of sorbitol, a form of carbohydrate, are among the worst beverages for children suffering from diarrhea. Prune, pear, and sweet cherry juice contain high levels of sorbitol, which is not absorbed fully by the body and can worsen diarrhea by producing watery stools. Fiber-filled foods increase stool clearance from the body, when the intent is just the opposite in a person recovering from diarrhea.

Lactase levels may temporarily decrease after a bout of diarrhea, which may make dairy foods intolerable for a time. This varies from person to person. Give small amounts of dairy products to your child along with other foods and monitor his dairy tolerance.

When Water Won't Do

Infants with diarrhea but no vomiting may tolerate breast milk or formula. But if they vomit after eating, they may require commercial oral electrolyte solutions. Same goes for older children who lose large amounts of fluid by throwing up or through diarrhea. In their many forms, the likes of Pedialyte, CeraLyte, and Infalyte provide fluid and electrolytes to prevent dehydration. Ask your pediatrician if your child requires such products.

SPITTING UP

Many babies are "spitters," but there's often little reason for concern, even when it looks like they spit back all the food they ate. Babies, especially ravenous ones, who gulp air and milk or formula while nursing or taking a bottle are likely to bring up some of the feeding when expelling the air. Spit-up is not usually problematic as long as your baby is happy and developing at the expected rate.

Nutritional Defense

You cannot shield your child from all germs, nor should you try. But you can beef up your youngster's immune system so that he gets sick less often and for less time. Here's how.

Breastfeed your baby. Nursing reduces the risk of upper respiratory and ear infections, as well as allergy and asthma.

Serve fruits and vegetables. They contain immunity-boosting phytochemicals.

Encourage healthy sleep habits. Keep kids on a sleep schedule. Limit television watching, and leave twenty to thirty minutes before bed for reading to your child to help them relax and ready them for sleep.

Supplement, don't substitute. In addition to a well-balanced diet, provide children with a daily multivitamin. It will help fill in any gaps in immunity-boosting nutrients, including vitamin C and the minerals iron and zinc.

Hold off on herbal supplements such as echinacea. Experts say there is no evidence that botanicals are safe for children.

Exercise as a family. Physical activity boosts the production of natural killer cells in adults, and there's little reason to think it won't do the same in children.

Wash your hands. Short of living in a plastic bubble, frequent hand washing is your best defense against germ transmission.

GASTROESOPHAGEAL REFLUX

Gastroesophageal reflux (GER) is more than spitting up. Think of GER as baby heartburn (which actually has nothing to do with the heart, by the way). After a baby eats, his stomach contents flow backwards into the esophagus, causing a burning sensation. A moderate case of GER can be treated by keeping baby in an upright position and feeding her smaller, more frequent meals. Offer your baby smaller amounts of formula or nurse more frequently so that you don't overload her tiny stomach. Don't wait until your baby is ravenous, since hungrier babies tend to gulp more air. Use gravity to your advantage and hold baby at a thirty- to forty-five-degree angle to keep air to a minimum. Don't use a car seat to achieve this with a bottle-fed baby. Very young babies are not able to sit up on their own. Propping up a newborn in a car seat actually causes slumping, creating pressure on baby's abdomen and making worse GER. More serious cases of GER may require medication and/or surgery to correct.

VOMITING

Vomiting is distressful for children and worrisome for parents. As in the case of diarrhea, dehydration is the primary threat to vomiting children. Deterring dehydration can prove challenging, particularly if a child's illness lasts for more than a day. Youngsters may have difficulty keeping down the fluid they need to meet their bodily needs plus make up for what they lose through vomit. Encourage slow and steady fluid intake. Even when your child brings up the fluid he swallowed, chances are he retained some of it. Try offering small amounts of water or crushed ice. If you think he can tolerate it, serve an ounce or so of diluted fruit juice every hour.

CONSTIPATION

If your child doesn't have a bowel movement every day, is she constipated? Not necessarily. Every youngster is unique, and so are his or her bowel habits.

Everyone gets constipated from time to time, particularly from age two years old and up. When it becomes a chronic condition, then there's cause for concern. Your child is constipated when he passes hard or dry stools that he cannot manage without straining or having pain during bowel movements.

The duo of fiber and fluid are a constipated child's best friend. Fiber-filled foods and fluid work together to alleviate constipation by increasing the size and softness of stools and making them easier to pass. That's one of the reasons why a diet rich in whole grains, fruits, and vegetables is so good for kids. Regular physical activity boosts blood circulation to the intestinal tract, which helps the system stay active and healthy. Do not give a child laxatives without your pediatrician's approval.

Some parents blame iron-fortified formula for their baby's infrequent bowel movements and mistakenly switch to low-iron infant formula. Iron may contribute to constipation in some people, but a baby doesn't need to move her bowels every day for optimum health. Furthermore, babies with deficient iron intake run the risk for health problems and developmental shortfalls.

FOOD AND BEHAVIOR: WHAT'S THE CONNECTION?

Your child is inattentive, impulsive, and naughty. Could be something he ate, or not. It's hard to define the exact connection between food and behavior. When your child is off the wall more often than not and you can't figure out why, it's easy to point a finger at his diet, although his behavior could be the result of inadequate sleep or stress of some kind. Is it fair to blame food for disobedience? Here's the lowdown.

The Usual Suspects

Sugar and caffeine produce energy jolts that can invite insolent behavior. Here's why, and how you can curb your child's consumption.

Caffeine

A can of caffeine-containing cola may make no difference in your behavior, but give the same amount to a preschooler and watch her take off. Caffeine is a central nervous system stimulant that can turn an otherwise obedient child into a whirling dervish who won't do what you ask of her and probably won't go to bed when you want her to, either. Caffeine causes wakefulness in children and may be anxiety producing in kids who don't consume it regularly. Children who consume caffeine on a daily basis may repeat their unruly behavior day after day and probably won't get the restful sleep they need, exacerbating the problem. See page 40 for more on cutting caffeine out of your child's life.

Iron

As part of red blood cells, iron is responsible for ferrying oxygen to your child's rapidly developing brain. It's also critical for overall brain function, including the ability for brain cells to communicate with each other. Low dietary iron levels impede your child's brain function and may reduce attentiveness and short-term memory. Iron-deficient children generally score lower on school achievement tests.

Sugar

Sugar provides an energy rush to a youngster's cells that can trigger hooting, hollering, and climbing of walls. Bouts of high-energy activity after simple sugar consumption are short lived, but serving sugary snacks throughout the day perpetuates inattention. The good news is that studies show that simple sugars, the kind found in cakes, cookies, ice cream, soda, fruit juice, and fruit drinks, produce no lasting effects on a youngster's learning or concentration. Nor is sugar the reason for Attention Deficit Hyperactivity Disorder (ADHD), a condition characterized by impulsiveness, inattention, distraction, and anxiety. Sugar is explained in detail beginning on page 13.

Attention Deficit Hyperactivity Disorder (ADHD)

Every child has his moments of restlessness and impulsivity. When preschoolers, more often boys, can't sit still; are disruptive during nursery school or kindergarten; and have trouble focusing on reading, writing, and other projects, it could be indicative of Attention Deficit Hyperactivity Disorder (ADHD), which affects one in twenty children. According to the U.S. Department of Health and Human Services, there are three kinds of ADHD; overactivity, inability to pay attention, and impulsiveness are common to all three kinds. Generally, a diagnosis of ADHD is made when symptoms are apparent before age seven and are chronic, lasting at least six months.

No one knows what causes ADHD, but experts say genetics probably plays a role. Other factors, including chemical exposure and viruses and situations that may impair brain development, such as problems during pregnancy or delivery, may also be at the root of some cases of ADHD.

Some parents say food additives, including artificial flavors, colors, and preservatives such as MSG, rank high on the list of agitators in children with ADHD. Perhaps the most notable eating regimen for hyperactive behavior was proposed in the 1970s by allergist Dr. Benjamin Feingold. Feingold claimed a diet free of artificial colors and flavors and devoid of produce with a high salicylate content, including apples, berries, tomatoes, oranges, green peppers, and tangerines, calmed children. Subsequent scientific studies using the Feingold diet could not support the claims for such dietary restrictions. That doesn't mean that certain food restrictions won't work to calm your youngster, however. It is possible for kids to be extra sensitive to certain foods or food ingredients. But don't make any dietary changes until you speak with your doctor about the suspected link between your child's diet and his behavior. Always work closely with a registered dietitian when attempting any elimination diet.

Chapter 16

Preparing
for
Pregnancy

Getting yourself ready
to have the healthiest
baby possible is the
greatest gift you could
give your future child.

—Nancy, *mother of four*

Another baby may seem unlikely right now, especially if you have a newborn. But if you are thinking about expanding your family, it's never too early to set the stage. Prospective parents who lead healthy lifestyles have a greater chance of having the brightest, healthiest babies. Even experienced moms and dads will learn from this chapter, since preconceptual advice often changes. Read on for more info on how prospective moms and dads should prepare for the baby in their future.

EXPECT THE BEST

Mom is largely responsible for her baby's well-being in the short term and in the long run. That seems reasonable, since she nurtures a developing baby inside of her body for nine months. Research published in the *American Journal of Clinical Nutrition* suggests that the risk for developing chronic conditions such as heart disease, high blood pressure, elevated cholesterol concentrations, and type 2 diabetes later in life is linked to the quality of Mom's diet during pregnancy, even when babies are born weighing within the acceptable range.

Some women are so busy with their other children that they ignore their own nutritional needs, grabbing high-fat food on the run, never sitting down to a decent meal, or skipping meals completely. Big mistake. Whether you conceive again or not, you must nourish yourself in order to take care of your family, never mind to prepare for another pregnancy. The following is food for thought for women in childbearing mode.

Achieve and maintain a healthy weight for at least three months before conceiving. Your baby's health is linked to your body weight when you become pregnant. Overweight mothers are at risk for complications during pregnancy, such as gestational diabetes and high blood pressure. They are also likelier to experience more difficult deliveries, which may involve cesarean section. Babies born to obese moms may have a harder time regulating their blood glucose level immediately after birth, requiring additional care.

Women who don't weigh enough can have problems, too. Conceiving a child may take longer. Once pregnant, underweight mothers are more likely to deliver premature babies and babies weighing under five and a half pounds (low-birth-weight babies). Low-birth-weight babies typically endure more health problems and developmental difficulties and may score lower on the Apgar test, too. The Apgar test determines the heart rate, breathing, muscle tone, responsiveness, and color of newborns at one and five minutes after birth.

Moms who put on extra pounds during a previous pregnancy may want to shed them before becoming pregnant again. That's OK, as long as you don't lose weight on unsafe diets and become underweight before conceiving.

Very low calorie diet programs that eliminate one or more of the five food groups are not for any woman. They may lead to speedy results, but fad diets do not work to keep off weight in the long term. Plus, very low calorie eating regimens are deficient in many of the nutrients that you must stockpile for your next baby, including calcium, iron, and zinc. Work on changing your diet for the better by eating from all of the five food groups every day, avoiding added fats and sweets, and putting on your daily menu three servings of dairy foods such as low-fat milk and yogurt.

Don't Drink Up

You're nearly ready to deliver, and you haven't had a glass of wine for months. What's the harm in a few drinks? Plenty. From six months on, your baby's brain is in a growth spurt that lasts until he's two. Even when you are days away from giving birth, a single, prolonged episode of exposure to alcohol (read: a few drinks) can kill millions of brain cells your baby needs for learning, memory, and thinking for the rest of his life.

Focus on folic acid. Folic acid is the man-made form of the B vitamin folate. In landmark research studies, folic acid helped prevent defects of the neural tube, including spina bifida. The neural tube is the part of a developing baby's body that becomes the spinal column and brain. But there's a catch. Folic acid provides peak protection from neural tube defects, including spina bifida, during the first twenty-eight days after conception, a time when many women don't realize that they are pregnant. That's why taking folic acid every day before conception is so important for helping to ensure a healthy baby with the brightest future possible.

The Centers for Disease Control and Prevention estimate that if every woman of childbearing age (between fourteen and fifty years of age) consumed 400 micrograms of daily folic acid, the rate of neural tube defects would drop by at least half. Does that mean that if you don't take supplemental folic acid your baby will be born with a neural tube deformity? Not necessarily, but folic acid at the right time during pregnancy significantly reduces the risk. Women should take full advantage of what folic acid has to offer.

Once you conceive, pregnancy requirements for folic acid increase to 600 micrograms daily. Folic acid helps prevent anemia during pregnancy. Preliminary research points to adequate folic acid intake as a way of warding off early miscarriage, too. Until you get a prescription for prenatal supplements from your doctor, continue taking an over-the-counter folic acid supplement. Prescription multivitamins provide enough folic acid for pregnancy, so cease taking any other dietary supplement once you begin the prescription pills. Your diet should also include foods filled with folate and folic acid, including fortified grains, lentils, spinach, wheat germ, orange juice, strawberries, asparagus, and broccoli.

Go slow on supplements. Taking a daily multivitamin is the easiest way for women to get the folic acid they need. Most multivitamins contain 400 micrograms of folic acid, along with a bevy of nutrients that can make up for small gaps in your diet and help you get into the best shape for pregnancy. Preliminary evidence suggests that daily multivitamins before pregnancy may also protect against cleft palate and could be slightly protective in warding off Down's syndrome.

Research published in the *American Journal of Epidemiology* has found that taking a multivitamin prior to conception significantly reduces the chances for having a baby with a heart defect. The authors of the study say it's difficult to pinpoint the exact effect of daily multivitamins on developing babies. Why? Because women who consume multivitamins may also eat healthier diets than women who don't. Even so, a daily multivitamin that provides about 100 percent of the DV for most nutrients won't harm you or your unborn child.

Keep food safe. You may not be pregnant yet, but you should know this. *Listeria moncytogenes*, a bacterium found in foods such as soft cheeses made with unpasteurized milk; deli meats; and undercooked meat, poultry, or seafood is harmful to an unborn child. When the infection is passed along from you to your developing baby, miscarriage is likely, and so are premature delivery and birth defects. For more on *Listeria monocytogenes*, see page 175.

Eating undercooked meat during pregnancy is the primary reason for *toxoplasmosis*, a parasite infection, according to the *British Medical Journal*. Toxoplasmosis can lead to brain damage in developing fetuses.

Give herbs the heave-ho. Researchers at Loma Linda University School of Medicine have found that St. John's wort, *Echinacea purpurea*, and *Ginkgo biloba* damaged both sperm and eggs, while Saw palmetto decreased sperm viability. Granted, the study was conducted in the laboratory using human sperm and hamster eggs, so it's hard to say what the results on a human pregnancy would be.

Indeed, other preliminary research indicates echinacea does not boost birth defect risk. However, it's important to note that herbal preparations have drug-like properties, despite being sold in the United States as dietary supplements. There is not a lot of scientific evidence that proves botanicals reduce fertility, harm sperm, or hurt a woman's eggs. On the other hand, there's no proof that they won't interfere with fertility, which is why any couple considering pregnancy should err on the side of safety.

Dump the (illicit) drugs. Recreational drugs during pregnancy have serious effects on an unborn child. For example, cocaine chokes off the flow of oxygen and nutrients to a developing baby. It increases the risk of miscarriage during the early months of pregnancy and triggers premature labor later on. Babies of women who use cocaine may die during the pregnancy or have a stroke that causes irreversible brain damage. Marijuana and other illicit drugs can have devastating effects, too.

Snub smoking. You're a smoker, but you don't puff away during pregnancy. That's admirable. Premature and low-birth-weight babies are but two of the results of smoking mothers. Moms who smoke also pass along a potent carcinogen to their unborn babies, which may lead to cancer later in life. In addition, babies born to moms who smoke are more likely to suffer from a cleft lip or palate, according to a study conducted by researchers at the University of Michigan Health System; the risk of this disfiguring facial birth defect increases with the number of cigarettes Mom smokes daily. If you're not pregnant and you're still smoking around your children, you should know that children of smokers are prone to developing asthma, a chronic condition they have for life. A study in the *Archives of Childhood Diseases* suggests that mothers who smoke are more likely to deliver colicky babies.

Cigarette smoking robs your body of vital nutrients such as vitamin C and wreaks havoc on long-term bone strength. Smokers are also sick more often and they may not be as tolerant of the physical demands of pregnancy the next time around, given their less-than-peak lung and heart function.

There's nothing good to say about smoking, which is why you should make every effort to quit as soon as possible to get in shape for your next baby and to protect family members from secondhand smoke.

Cut the caffeine. The relationship between caffeine and conception is cloudy. One study published in the *American Journal of Epidemiology* found that women who consumed more than 300 milligrams of caffeine daily had to wait more than a year before being able to conceive a child. A study appearing in the *New England Journal of Medicine* indicated that as little as 100 milligrams of caffeine daily increases miscarriage risk. Whatever the case, it's a good idea to examine, and possibly, curb your caffeine intake starting now, since you should consume very little caffeine during pregnancy, if any at all. Caffeine hangs around longer in a pregnant woman's body than in her nonpregnant counterpart's, and could negatively affect your baby when consumed in large quantities. See page 40 for more on caffeine.

Avoid alcohol. You know that drinking during pregnancy is out of the question, but drinking while you're trying to conceive may be a bad idea, too. The American Academy of Pediatrics (AAP) advises against consuming alcohol while trying to conceive. Every year, more than fifty thousand babies are born in the United States with some degree of alcohol-related damage, according to the March of Dimes. Alcohol deprives developing cells of oxygen, hampering your unborn child's growth. Alcohol's effects during pregnancy are irreparable. The March of Dimes says children exposed to alcohol while in the womb wind up with a variety of deficiencies ranging from mental and physical retardation to lower IQ scores, aggressive behavior, and inability to pay attention in the classroom once they are in school.

Determine drug safety. You probably don't think twice about the medications you use regularly, but when pregnancy is in the offing, you'll want to give your medicine chest the once over. For example, the prescription acne medication Accutane (isotretinoin) has been found to cause birth defects, according to the Centers for Disease Control and Prevention. Ask your doctor about the safety of any prescription and over-the-counter medications you use on a regular basis or are planning to take any time soon.

Cancel the chemicals. Common household products such as solvents and pesticides contain chemicals that can harm unborn children. When cleaning or renovating any area of your house, make sure it's well ventilated. Once you become pregnant, avoid remodeling projects and don't handle pesticides.

Check your cholesterol. You're young, so why have your blood cholesterol concentration checked before conceiving? Because it could affect the health of your future son or daughter. Elevated blood cholesterol levels in moms-to-be may increase the risk of abnormally high blood pressure during pregnancy, a condition called preeclampsia. Uncontrolled high blood pressure can lead to premature delivery and seizures. And a study in *The Lancet* suggests that women who enter pregnancy with an elevated blood cholesterol level increase the risk, and speed the progression of, heart disease in their child. It seems Mom's blood cholesterol levels are tied to Junior's propensity for fatty streaks. Fatty streaks mark the beginnings of clogged arteries that can result in heart disease. Before trying for another child, have a thorough physical examination that takes into account your blood cholesterol level. If your cholesterol is high, seek the guidance of a registered dietitian to help you follow a healthy preconception diet designed to lower blood cholesterol concentrations.

For Folate, Go for the (Enriched) Grain

Folic acid, the form that matters most when thwarting birth defects, does not occur naturally in foods to any appreciable extent. Thanks to supplementation required by law, cereal, bread, and pasta supply significant amounts of added folic acid. Not all grains are fortified, however. Only enriched grains are required by law to contain folic acid. That means that folic acid may be missing from your morning coffee-shop bagel. Since food labels do not appear on those items, it's next to impossible to figure out if they provide the folic acid you need.

Even with food labels, figuring folic acid levels can be challenging for a number of reasons. Manufacturers are allowed to use the term *folate* on the Nutrition Facts panel to describe the folate or folic acid level in foods. Folate is folic acid's naturally occurring counterpart. Folate is absorbed by the body at half the rate of folic acid. How do you know that folic acid is present? Read the ingredient list.

Then there's the DV to consider. Here's how to figure what you get from food. If two ounces of dry pasta provide 25 percent of the DV, it means that serving supplies 100 micrograms of folic acid. That's because the DV for folic acid is 400 micrograms.

Finally, some enriched grains do not bother to post folic acid content on the Nutrition Facts panel, which is why you must be a label sleuth and study the ingredients. Products containing enriched flour list folic acid as one of its ingredients. Not all grains are enriched, however. That means that the bread, pasta, rice, cereal, and other grains you eat on a regular basis may not supply folic acid.

Food	Amount	Folic Acid (micrograms)
Ready-to-eat cereal	1 ounce	100–400
Pasta	1 cup cooked	100–120
Rice	1 cup cooked	88
Wheat germ	2 tablespoons	56
Waffle, frozen	1 4-inch waffle	27
Whole wheat bread	1 slice	20

Boost baby's brain power. Women planning to conceive should stock up on DHA. DHA is a polyunsaturated fat that's concentrated in the cells of baby's brain and eyes. Some experts say high levels of DHA may make your baby smarter and able to see better. Women can stockpile DHA for pregnancy by regularly eating foods such as fish, or eggs with added omega-3s. Vegetarians who eschew all animal foods would do well to consume foods laden with linolenic acid, a fat that the body can convert to DHA. See pages 57 and 58 for more on food sources of DHA and linolenic acid.

All fish are not equally beneficial, however. In fact, some are downright detrimental. The FDA says pregnant women, women in the childbearing years, and nursing moms should not consume swordfish, shark, tilefish, or king mackerel. These large ocean fish may have concentrations of mercury, which is toxic to baby's developing nervous system. Women can safely eat 12 ounces a week of cooked shellfish, canned fish, smaller ocean fish, or farm-raised fish. Fish caught out of rivers and streams, especially in the Great Lakes region, are more likely to contain pesticides and polychlorinated biphenyls (PCBs). PCBs are no longer produced in the United States, but they continue to contaminate many rivers and lakes. Your body can store PCBs. Ingesting them before pregnancy (and during) may compromise a child's brain development, resulting in persistent problems with memory and cognition. Sport fishermen should always check the state fishing advisory to see if their favorite fishing grounds are contaminated. See the EPA's online database at *http://fish.rti.org* and the EPA's Consumption Advisory site at *www.epa.gov.ost/fish* to get started.

Timing Is Everything

It may not be possible, but an article in the *New England Journal of Medicine* suggests that women should wait at least eighteen months after giving birth to get pregnant again. Why? Pregnancy and birth are taxing. Bearing children in quick succession puts added strain on your bodily stores of calcium and iron, never mind dragging on your energy level, especially if you're breastfeeding.

Iron it out. Have a history of iron deficiency? Check out your blood-iron levels before embarking on another pregnancy. You may not have any outward signs of low iron stores, but that could change once pregnancy begins. Pregnancy is a drag on iron levels, largely because of the increase in blood volume that occurs mostly during the first trimester. Iron is part of blood cells, which are needed in abundance to ferry oxygen to your developing baby. Adequate iron also ensures proper nervous system growth during pregnancy. Iron is part of the myelination process, during which the body wraps nerve fibers in myelin, which promotes effective communication throughout your child's nervous system.

Lose the lead. Lead disrupts a child's normal brain development. Dwellings constructed before 1986 may have plumbing that contains lead that can leach into tap water. Copper pipes are not without their pitfalls, since they may be joined by lead solder.

Lead builds up in Mom's body, and she can transmit it to her developing baby during pregnancy. Decrease your lifetime lead exposure by avoiding imported cosmetics like kohl and Surma and staying away from calcium supplements made from potentially lead-laden bonemeal or dolomite. All family members should avoid chipping lead paint, and the lead dust produced by home renovations or refinishing furniture. Never stay in your home when repair or renovation of lead paint surfaces is being done; and don't bring family members back into the home unless it's been properly cleaned. See "Get the Lead Out," page 60 for more information.

Making the Most of Multivitamins

Multivitamins offer inexpensive protection against birth defects and help shore up nutrient stores that may be in short supply when preparing for pregnancy. Which multi is best? Cut through the confusion with these buying tips.

Utilize USP. The United States Pharmacopoeia (USP) is an independent group of health experts. Look for the USP stamp of approval on supplement labels to guarantee that your multivitamin will dissolve properly in the body. Dissolution is necessary for nutrient absorption.

Note the date. Nutrients don't last forever. Choose supplements with the date furthest in the future.

Go generic. Buy a famous brand knock-off to save money while getting the nutrients you need. Supplements need not be expensive or sport fancy labeling terms like *chelated* and *stress formula* to be effective.

Drink up. Take pills with meals or substantial snacks and plenty of water.

Store supplements in a cool, dry place. Humidity and light destroy nutrients.

Avoid interference. Avoid mixing your iron-containing multivitamin with calcium supplements. Iron and calcium compete for absorption in your digestive tract.

See the dentist. Don't put off dental health, especially if you're planning a pregnancy. Going into pregnancy with a clean bill of health from your dentist is key to having a healthy child. Mouth infections such as gingivitis can result in a chain of events leading to premature delivery, according to a study at the University of Alabama School of Dentistry. Here's why. Hormonal surges in early pregnancy produce puffy and tender gums that are more vulnerable to the bacteria that live in your mouth. The trouble starts when gums become inflamed as a result of germs. Your body responds to a mouth infection in much the same way it acts to trigger labor: by producing more prostaglandins and cytokines. When prostaglandins and cytokines make their way into amniotic fluid, they jump-start labor and may cause a baby to be delivered before his due date.

In My Experience
Don't Get Caught Off Guard

At work and at home, women plan so many things that they are easily lulled into thinking they can always control when they become pregnant. Don't be so sure. More than half of all pregnancies in the United States are unexpected, according to the Centers for Disease Control and Prevention. I am living proof of that. I got caught off guard not once, but twice. My second and third pregnancies were surprises, of sorts. Tom and I wanted more children after Hayley, but we just didn't think that I would get pregnant at those particular times. That's why it's imperative to follow the expert advice that women in their childbearing years who are capable of becoming pregnant (yes, even if you are using birth control) consume 400 micrograms of folic acid daily. You just never know.

FOR MEN ONLY: THE FATHER FACTOR

Your baby's well-being is not just the mom's responsibility. Dad's contribution to a healthy baby begins well before the moment of conception.

Sperm are vulnerable to toxins and to a man's unhealthy lifestyle habits. When sperm with damaged genetic material manage to fertilize an egg, it often spells trouble for a developing baby, leading to stillbirth, birth defects, learning disabilities, and childhood cancers, according to the March of Dimes. Here's how to keep your sperm health up to speed.

Curb the chemicals. Certain occupations are particularly harmful to a man's fertility. Autoworkers, agricultural workers, painters, and men working in chemical manufacturing are among those at risk for exposure to reproductive hazards such as lead, the pesticide kepone, benzene, anesthetic gases, and ionizing radiation. These substances produce a range of harmful effects in humans, including reduced sperm counts, genetic damage, miscarriage, and birth defects; dozens more materials can cause reproductive problems in animals.

Snuff the butts. When men smoke, their sperm quality suffers, and sperm count is lower. They may also suffer from a lower sex drive and have sex less frequently than their nonsmoking peers. Maybe that's why when men smoke, but not women, it can take a couple longer to conceive a baby. According to the March of Dimes, smoking ten cigarettes a day lowers the number of sperm men produce. One study suggests that when men smoke before their partners conceive, they are 20 percent more likely to have a child who goes on to develop brain cancer, lymphoma, and leukemia.

Chances are, you already have at least one child at home, which is one of the reasons to give up smoking now. The other is your future child. Babies born to women whose husband or male partner smokes are at risk for being underweight and vulnerable to an array of health problems now and in the future.

Avoid alcohol. The link between moderate drinking and the well-being of your future baby is murky, but experts do know this: alcoholic males produce sperm with defects that hamper their ability to fertilize the woman's egg. Limit alcohol to two drinks a day or less, as long as you have no trouble handling it or do not operate a car or heavy machinery after drinking. A drink is defined as one of the following: 12 ounces of regular beer, 5 ounces of wine, or 1½ ounces of 80-proof distilled spirits.

Keep cool. If you're trying to conceive, forget about regular trips to the hot tub. Prolonged heat is sperm's enemy. Sperm thrive at moderate temperatures. Steaming water in hot tubs suppresses sperm count, as does wearing tight workout gear to pedal long distances on your bike. Don't worry about your underwear, however. Both boxers and briefs are equally conducive to higher sperm counts.

Drop the drugs. Prescription and over-the-counter medications, including certain antibiotics and ulcer drugs, may impair a man's fertility. Consult your doctor or pharmacist about the medications you take regularly or are planning to use. The bodybuilding supplements DHEA and androstenedione depress sperm production; large doses of muscle-building testosterone can render a man permanently infertile. Illegal drugs lower your chances of having a healthy baby, too. Marijuana and cocaine use depresses sperm numbers. Even worse, cocaine can adhere to sperm. Should a cocaine-containing sperm fertilize an egg and produce a baby, there could be serious health repercussions.

Viva vitamin C. Vitamin C is necessary for vigorous sperm. One small study done at the University of California at Berkeley found that men deprived of vitamin C produced faulty sperm with damaged genetic material that could result in birth defects and chronic illness, such as cancer, should they ever fertilize an egg. When men took 60 milligrams of vitamin C every day for four weeks—about the amount typically found in a regular multivitamin pill—sperm damage dropped off. Men can get enough vitamin C by eating at least five servings of fruits and vegetables daily, especially if one of the choices is a citrus fruit. Smoking reduces levels of vitamin C in the body. Male smokers require at least 125 milligrams of daily vitamin C to counteract cigarettes' effects on vitamin C levels.

Wait a while. Sperm health does not improve overnight. It takes ten to twelve weeks to produce top-notch sperm. After making changes for the better, take some time before trying for a baby. It will be well worth the wait.

Chapter 17

Nutritious,

Delicious

Family Fare

Fluffy Pancakes

Serves 4 (Makes 12 pancakes.)

Add fresh or frozen blueberries, dried cranberries, or raisins to boost the fiber in these calcium-packed kid-favorites.

1 cup plain nonfat yogurt
1 large egg
1 cup pancake mix

In a bowl, combine yogurt and egg. Mix well. Add pancake mix and blend just to combine. Lightly oil or spray a nonstick pan or griddle. Ladle out 2 tablespoons batter per pancake. When edges are firm, turn pancakes and cook 1 minute more. Serve immediately.

Serving size: 3 pancakes.

Per serving: 173 calories, 8 grams protein, 2 grams fat, 30 grams carbohydrate, 1 gram fiber, 62 milligrams cholesterol, 1 milligram iron, 545 milligrams sodium, 272 milligrams calcium, 0 vitamin C, 1 milligram zinc, 44 micrograms folate.

QUICK BREADS

Cheesy Corn Muffins

Makes 18.

Each muffin supplies nearly as much
protein as an ounce of meat or fish.

1 cup 1% low-fat milk
1 cup low-fat cottage cheese
2 eggs
½ cup packed shredded cheddar cheese (about 2 ounces)
2 8½-ounce packages corn muffin mix

Preheat oven to 400°F. Line 12 standard-size muffin cups with paper liners. Combine milk, cottage cheese, and eggs in large bowl. Use electric mixer to blend on medium speed for one to two minutes. Stir in cheddar cheese, then stir in corn muffin mix until just blended. Do not overmix.

Spoon batter into prepared muffin cups, dividing equally. Bake about 13–15 minutes, or until muffins are light brown on top and tester inserted into center comes out clean. Let muffins cool to room temperature.

Serving size: 1 muffin.

Per serving: 143 calories, 5 grams protein, 5 grams fat, 20 grams carbohydrate, 1 gram fiber, 29 milligrams cholesterol, 0 iron, 290 milligrams sodium, 93 milligrams calcium, 0 vitamin C, 0 zinc, 42 micrograms folate.

Shaken, Baked Chicken Nuggets
Serves 4–8.
My kids love to help prepare this dish.

½ cup all-purpose flour
¼ cup grated Parmesan cheese
1 cup seasoned bread crumbs
¾ cup fat-free buttermilk
1 pound boneless, skinless chicken breast, cut into small
    chunks or strips
1 tablespoon canola or olive oil

Preheat oven to 400°F. Rinse chicken and pat dry with paper towels. Measure flour into a resealable 1-gallon plastic bag. Do the same for the bread crumbs in a separate 1-gallon plastic bag. (You may want to use more bags if you are preparing this with more than one child.) Pour buttermilk into a shallow bowl.

Add chicken pieces one at a time to the flour bag and shake until coated. Dip each piece of chicken into buttermilk, covering thoroughly, and letting extra buttermilk drain off. Then place each chicken chunk one at a time into the bread crumb bag and shake to cover.

Grease baking sheet with oil. Place coated chicken pieces on baking sheet. Cook for 5 minutes. Flip and cook for another 5 minutes, or until done.

Serving size: About 2 ounces.

Per serving: 175 calories, 17 grams protein, 4 grams fat, 17 grams carbohydrate, 1 gram fiber, 35 milligrams cholesterol, 1 milligram iron, 485 milligrams sodium, 272 milligrams calcium, 0 vitamin C, 1 milligram zinc, 21 micrograms folate.

ENTREES AND VEGETABLES

Mac and Cheese

Makes 4 cups.

As quick and easy as the boxed versions.

8 ounces uncooked small macaroni such as elbow or orzo

¼ cup 1% low-fat milk

1 tablespoon margarine

4 ounces cheddar cheese, grated (or any other hard cheese)

Cook pasta according to directions. After cooking and draining pasta, return to saucepan. Add milk, margarine, and cheese. Stir until melted.

Serving size: ½ cup.

Per serving: 178 calories, 7 grams protein, 7 grams fat, 22 grams carbohydrate, 1 gram fiber, 15 milligrams cholesterol, 1 milligram iron, 110 milligrams sodium, 117 milligrams calcium, 0 vitamin C, 1 milligram zinc, 128 micrograms folate.

Beef Pouch Potatoes

Serves 6.

Kids think it's cool to eat from a pouch.
Open pouches slowly after cooking and let them
sit for a few minutes before serving.

6 sheets (12" square) heavy-duty aluminum foil
4 medium potatoes, sliced ¼-inch thick
16 ounces sirloin steak
12 ounces prepared beef gravy
2 cups frozen peas
1 medium red bell pepper, cut into strips
1 teaspoon salt
1 teaspoon pepper, if desired

Heat oven to 450°F. In medium bowl, mix all ingredients; divide equally among the aluminum foil sheets. Place mixture on one side of the foil squares. Seal each pouch by folding one side over another, but leave room for heat to circulate inside pouches. Place on baking sheet and bake in center of oven for 35 minutes. When done, open slowly, allowing steam to escape. Cool before serving to children.

Serving size: 1 pouch.

Per serving: 406 calories, 29 grams protein, 12 grams fat, 45 grams carbohydrate, 5 grams fiber, 67 milligrams cholesterol, 5 milligrams iron, 110 milligrams sodium, 117 milligrams calcium, 74 milligrams vitamin C, 15 milligrams zinc, 8 micrograms folate.

Cream of Broccoli Soup

Serves 8.

A colorful and delicious way to disguise a healthy food.

6 cups broccoli florets or
  2 10-ounce packages frozen broccoli
1 cup chicken broth
2 tablespoons margarine
2 tablespoons all-purpose flour
$\frac{1}{2}$ teaspoon dried thyme
$\frac{1}{2}$ teaspoon salt
2 cups 1% low-fat milk

Cook broccoli until crisp-tender. In blender or food processor, combine broccoli and chicken broth. Cover and blend until smooth, about a minute or so.

Melt margarine in a medium saucepan. Stir in flour, thyme, and salt. Add milk and stir. Cook and stir until slightly thickened and bubbly. Cook 1 minute more and stir in broccoli mixture. Cook until heated through, stirring constantly.

Serving size: 1 cup.

Per serving: 81 calories, 4 grams protein, 4 grams fat, 8 grams carbohydrate, 2 grams fiber, 3 milligrams cholesterol, 1 milligram iron, 325 milligrams sodium, 110 milligrams calcium, 62 milligrams vitamin C, 0 milligram zinc, 51 micrograms folate.

Mushroom Frittata

Serves 6.

A speedy supper or brunch item.
Substitute zucchini and tomato for the mushrooms.

5 eggs
salt and pepper, to taste, if desired
1 teaspoon dried basil
1 cup low-fat cottage cheese
5 tablespoons grated Parmesan cheese
2 tablespoons canola oil
1 cup sliced mushrooms

In a medium bowl, beat eggs lightly with salt, pepper, basil, and oregano.

Stir in cottage cheese and half the Parmesan cheese.

In a 12-inch nonstick skillet, lightly sauté mushrooms in the canola oil until soft.

Pour in egg mixture and sprinkle with remaining Parmesan cheese. Cook over medium-low heat until eggs are well set on bottom of pan, about 15 minutes. Cut into wedges and serve hot.

Serving size: ⅙ of the frittata.

Per serving: 164 calories, 13 grams protein, 11 grams fat, 3 grams carbohydrate, 0 fiber, 209 milligrams cholesterol, 1 milligram iron, 148 milligrams sodium, 101 milligrams calcium, 0 vitamin C, 1 milligram zinc, 29 micrograms folate.

ENTREES AND VEGETABLES

Stuffed Potato

Serves 2.

This spud's a winner with kids.
Each portion provides one and a half vegetable servings.

1 large potato, baked
½ cup low-fat cottage cheese
1 cup steamed vegetables such as broccoli
and red bell pepper, coarsely chopped
¼ cup sharp cheddar cheese, grated

Preheat oven to 425°F.

Slice baked potato lengthwise. Carefully scoop out potato, leaving about ¼-inch of pulp inside the shell. Mash the potato in a medium mixing bowl.

Mix in the cottage cheese, onion powder, black pepper, and cooked vegetables. Place potato shells on baking sheet. Spoon mixture back into potato shells.

Top with cheddar cheese. Bake for 10–15 minutes or until cheese melts.

Serving size: One potato.

Per serving: 223 calories, 14 grams protein, 6 grams fat, 30 grams carbohydrate, 3 grams fiber, 18 milligrams cholesterol, 2 milligrams iron, 123 milligrams sodium, 163 milligrams calcium, 54 milligrams vitamin C, 1 milligram zinc, 45 micrograms folate.

Mashed Sweet Potatoes

Serves 6.

The entire family will enjoy this carotenoid-containing side dish.

3 medium sweet potatoes, peeled and cut into 1" cubes
3 tablespoons brown sugar, firmly packed (optional)
¼ cup orange juice
1 tablespoon margarine

Cook sweet potatoes until soft. Mash with brown sugar, orange juice, and margarine.

Serving size: ½ cup.

Per serving (made with brown sugar): 137 calories, 2 grams protein, 2 grams fat, 29 grams carbohydrate, 3 grams fiber, 0 cholesterol, 0 iron, 36 milligrams sodium, 26 milligrams calcium, 23 milligrams vitamin C, 2 milligrams zinc, 16 micrograms folate.

Chicken Pot Pie

Serves 6.

*A lot easier and faster to make
than it appears. Use turkey for a change.*

Filling:
2 cups frozen or fresh crinkle-cut carrots
$\frac{1}{2}$ cup chicken broth
$1\frac{1}{2}$ cups 1% low-fat milk
$\frac{1}{4}$ cup all-purpose flour
1 teaspoon dried sage leaves
1 tablespoon margarine
$\frac{1}{2}$ teaspoon salt
2 cups cubed cooked chicken
$1\frac{1}{2}$ cups frozen or fresh peas

Topping:
1 cup all-purpose flour
1 teaspoon baking powder
$\frac{1}{2}$ teaspoon salt
$\frac{1}{8}$ teaspoon baking soda
2 tablespoons margarine
$\frac{1}{2}$ cup fat-free buttermilk

(continued)

Heat oven to 400°F. Spray a 2-quart casserole with vegetable spray. In large saucepan, combine carrots and broth and bring to a boil. Cover and reduce heat, simmering for 2–3 minutes or until carrots are crisp-tender.

For filling: In a small bowl, whisk together milk and flour and blend well. Stir milk mixture, sage, margarine, and salt into carrot mixture. Bring to a boil, stirring constantly. Boil for 1 minute longer. Stir in chicken and peas. Pour entire filling mixture into prepared casserole dish.

For topping: In medium bowl, combine first 4 ingredients and stir. Cut in the margarine until mixture resembles coarse meal. Add buttermilk, stirring well to mix. Drop by teaspoons onto chicken mixture, covering it entirely.

Bake for 25–30 minutes, or until biscuits are golden brown.

Serving size: ⅙ of the pie.

Per serving: 320 calories, 22 grams protein, 11 grams fat, 33 grams carbohydrate, 3 grams fiber, 45 milligrams cholesterol, 3 milligrams iron, 857 milligrams sodium, 180 milligrams calcium, 9 milligrams vitamin C, 2 milligrams zinc, 37 micrograms folate.

Berry Smoothie

Serves 2.

Use your favorite berry to concoct this colorful treat.

1 cup 1% low-fat milk (use full fat for kids under two)
¾ cup berries, such as strawberries
1 teaspoon sugar
½ teaspoon vanilla extract
3 ice cubes, or about ½ cup crushed ice

Combine all ingredients in blender or food processor. Blend on high speed for 2–3 minutes, or until frothy. Pour into tall glass. Serve immediately.

> **Serving size:** ½ of the recipe.
>
> **Per serving (made with 1% low-fat milk):** 82 calories, 4 grams protein, 1 gram fat, 13 grams carbohydrate, 0 fiber, 5 milligrams cholesterol, 0 iron, 62 milligrams sodium, 159 milligrams calcium, 24 milligrams vitamin C, 0 zinc, 16 micrograms folate.

Pineapple Orange Smoothie

Serves 2.

*A great way to sneak in a fruit serving
and get calcium in the bargain.*

8 ounces calcium-fortified orange juice

¼ cup pineapple chunks, drained

¼ cup low-fat vanilla yogurt (full-fat for kids under two)

Combine all ingredients in a blender or food processor. Blend on high speed for 2–3 minutes, or until frothy. Serve immediately.

Serving size: ½ of the recipe.

Per serving (made with low-fat yogurt): 97 calories, 1 gram protein, 0 fat, 20 grams carbohydrate, 0 fiber, 2 milligrams cholesterol, 0 iron, 26 milligrams sodium, 203 milligrams calcium, 39 milligrams vitamin C, 0 zinc, 4 micrograms folate.

BEVERAGES

Cantaloupe Cooler

Serves 2.

Fortified juice packs calcium into this dairy-free beverage.

1 cup cubed cantaloupe
½ cup calcium-fortified orange juice
2 teaspoons honey
¼ teaspoon vanilla extract

Combine all ingredients in a blender or food processor. Blend on high speed for 2–3 minutes, or until frothy. Serve immediately.

Serving size: ½ of the recipe.

Per serving: 80 calories, 1 gram protein, 0 fat, 19 grams carbohydrate, 0 fiber, 0 cholesterol, 0 iron, 11 milligrams sodium, 85 milligrams calcium, 52 milligrams vitamin C, 0 zinc, 14 micrograms folate.

No-Bake Nut Butter Crunchies

Makes 16 1-inch balls.

These candy alternatives are fun to make and fun to eat. And they are a surprising source of high-quality protein, and calcium, too.

$\frac{1}{2}$ cup almond butter (or peanut butter)

$\frac{1}{2}$ cup honey

1 teaspoon vanilla extract

$\frac{3}{4}$ cup powdered milk

$\frac{2}{3}$ cup crispy rice cereal

Blend together almond butter, honey, and vanilla. Add powdered milk and cereal and blend well. Roll into balls.

Serving size: 2 balls.

Per serving: 230 calories, 6 grams protein, 11 grams fat, 28 grams carbohydrate, 1 gram fiber, 12 milligrams cholesterol, 1 milligram iron, 132 milligrams sodium, 146 milligrams calcium, 2 milligrams vitamin C, 1 milligram zinc, 26 micrograms folate.

Blueberry Cobbler
Serves 8.
*A nutritious way to use one of nature's
most potent disease-fighting fruits.*

Filling:
> 4 cups fresh or frozen blueberries
> 1½ tablespoons cornstarch
> ¼ cup water
> ⅔ cup sugar

Topping:
> 1 cup all-purpose flour
> ¼ cup sugar
> 1 teaspoon baking powder
> ½ teaspoon ground cinnamon
> 3 tablespoons margarine
> ¼ cup 1% low-fat milk
> 1 egg, beaten

(continued)

Heat oven to 400°F.

For filling, combine sugar, water, and cornstarch in a medium saucepan. Stir in blueberries. Cook until thickened, stirring constantly.

For topping, combine flour, sugar, baking powder, and if desired, cinnamon. Cut in margarine until the mixture resembles coarse crumbs. Combine egg and milk in a small bowl. Add to flour mixture, stirring just to moisten.

Transfer filling to a 2-quart rectangular baking dish. Drop about 12 mounds or so of topping over filling. Bake for 25 minutes or until a toothpick inserted into topping comes out clean.

Serving size: ⅛ of the recipe.

Per serving: 243 calories, 3 grams protein, 6 grams fat, 46 grams carbohydrate, 3 grams fiber, 31 milligrams cholesterol, 1 milligram iron, 125 milligrams sodium, 57 milligrams calcium, 2 milligrams vitamin C, 0 zinc, 13 micrograms folate.

Trail Mix*

Serves 3.

Don't let the high fat levels in this snack throw you.
With its fiber and iron, this mixture beats candy by a mile.

⅓ cup raisins or dried cranberries
⅓ cup chocolate chips
⅓ cup chopped almonds or other nuts**

Mix together ingredients in a small bowl.

Note: This snack is inappropriate for children ages four and under because the ingredients can cause choking.

**Roasted soy nuts, which contain about half the fat of nuts, may be used instead.

Serving size: ⅓ cup.

Per serving: 231 calories, 12 grams protein, 18 grams fat, 20 grams carbohydrate, 5 grams fiber, 0 cholesterol, 6 milligrams iron, 5 milligrams sodium, 30 milligrams calcium, 1 milligram vitamin C, 1 milligram zinc, 13 micrograms folate.

Hummus

Makes 1 cup.

This is a speedy, lower fat version of store-bought varieties.

1 tablespoon sesame oil
1 15-ounce can garbanzo beans, drained and rinsed
1 tablespoon lemon juice
$\frac{1}{2}$ teaspoon salt
$\frac{1}{2}$ teaspoon ground cumin (optional)
$\frac{1}{3}$ cup fresh parsley, minced

Puree until smooth in food processor all the ingredients except parsley. Stir in parsley. Serve with low-fat crackers, toasted pita bread, or fresh vegetables.

Serving size: 2 tablespoons.

Per serving: 79 calories, 3 grams protein, 2 grams fat, 12 grams carbohydrate, 2 grams fiber, 0 cholesterol, 1 milligram iron, 146 milligrams sodium, 17 milligrams calcium, 3 milligrams vitamin C, 1 milligram zinc, 36 micrograms folate.

DESSERTS AND SNACKS

Chewy Granola Bars
Makes 18.

Prepare a double batch and freeze some.

¼ cup margarine
¼ cup canola oil
¾ cup brown sugar
1 egg
1 teaspoon vanilla extract
1 cup all-purpose flour
½ teaspoon baking soda
½ teaspoon salt
¼ cup wheat germ
2¾ cups rolled oats
¾ cup chopped dates
¾ cup dried cranberries

Preheat oven to 350°F. Lightly grease a 9" × 13" × 2" baking pan. In a mixing bowl, cream together margarine, oil, and brown sugar. Add egg and vanilla and continue to beat on high speed for a minute or two. Sift together flour, baking soda, and salt; stir in wheat germ. Add to creamed mixture and mix well. Stir in rolled oats and dried fruit. Press evenly in pan.

Bake for 20 minutes or until lightly brown. Slice into bars.

Serving size: 1 bar.

Per serving: 203 calories, 4 grams protein, 8 grams fat, 31 grams carbohydrate, 3 grams fiber, 12 milligrams cholesterol, 1 milligram iron, 137 milligrams sodium, 21 milligrams calcium, 0 vitamin C, 1 milligram zinc, 45 micrograms folate.

Chapter 18

Resources

ASTHMA AND ALLERGY

Allergy and Asthma Network/Mothers
of Asthmatics, Inc.
800-878-4403

American Academy of Allergy, Asthma
and Immunology
800-822-2762
www.aaaai.org

American College of Allergy and
Asthma
800-842-7777
www.allergy.mcg.edu

Asthma and Allergy Foundation of
America
800-7-ASTHMA (727-8462)
www.aafa.org

Celiac Disease Foundation
818-990-2354

The Food Allergy Network
800-929-4040
www.foodallergy.org

JAMA Asthma Information Center
www.ama-assn.org/asthma

National Digestive Diseases
Information Clearinghouse
301-654-3810

BEHAVIOR

The Center for Mental Health Services
800-789-2647
www.mentalhealth.org

National Attention Deficit Disorder
Association
847-432-ADDA
www.add.org

United States Department of Health
and Human Services
877-696-6775
www.hhs.gov

BREASTFEEDING

Academy of Breastfeeding Medicine
913-541-9077
www.bfmed.org

Breast Pumps:
Medela 800-TELL-YOU
Ameda-Egnell 800-323-4060

International Lactation Consultants
Organization
919-787-5181
www.ilca.org

La Leche League
Help Line: 800-525-3243
www.lalecheleague.org

Nursing Mothers Advisory Council
www.nursingmoms.net

FOOD SAFETY

Centers for Disease Control and
Prevention
800-232-4674
www.cdc.gov

Environmental Protection Agency
202-260-2090
www.epa.gov/safewater

Food Safety and Inspection Service
202-720-7943
www.fsis.usda.gov

Government Food Safety Information
www.foodsafety.gov

International Bottled Water
Association
703-683-5213
www.bottledwater.org

International Food Information
Council
202-296-6540
www.ificinfo.health.org

Mothers and Others for a Livable
Planet
888-ECO-INFO
www.mothers.org

National Food Safety Database
www.foodsafety.org

National Sanitation Foundation
800-NSF-MARK
www.nsf.org

Organic Consumers Association
218-226-4164
www.purefood.org

Organic Trade Association
413-774-7511
www.ota.com

Union of Concerned Scientists
617-547-5552
www.ucsusa.org

United States Department of
Agriculture's Meat
and Poultry Hotline for Consumers
800-535-4555 (In the Washington,
D.C. area, call 202-720-3333.)

GENERAL NUTRITION AND HEALTH

American Academy of Pediatric
Dentistry
www.aapd.org

American Academy of Pediatrics
800-433-4000
www.aap.org

American Cancer Society
800-ACS-2345
www.cancer.org

American Dental Association
312-440-2500
www.ada.org

American Dental Hygienists
Association
312-440-8900
www.adha.org

American Diabetes Association
800-232-3472
www.diabetes.org

American Dietetic Association
800-877-1600
www.eatright.org (also provides free
referral to a registered dietitian in
your area)

American Heart Association
800-AHA-USA1
www.americanheart.org

American Institute for Cancer
Research
800-843-8114
www.aicr.org

National Institutes of Health
www.nih.gov

National Osteoporosis Foundation
202-223-2226
www.nof.org

The President's Council on Physical
Fitness and Sports
202-690-9000
www.fitness.gov

Produce for Better Health Foundation
302-738-7100
www.pma.com/5aday

United States Department of
Agriculture
202-418-2312
www.usda.gov

United States Food and Drug
Administration/Center
for Food Safety and Applied Nutrition
800-INFO-FDA
www.cfsan.fda.gov

Also:
www.family.go.com
www.freshstarts.com
www.kidfood.org
www.kidshealth.org
www.nutritionexplorations.com

HERBAL MEDICINE

The American Botanical Council
512-926-4900
www.herbalgram.org

National Center for Complementary
and Alternative Medicine
888-644-6226
www.nccam.nih.gov

PREGNANCY AND FERTILITY

American College of Obstetricians and
Gynecologists
800-762-2264
www.acog.org

American Society for Reproductive Medicine
205-978-5000
www.asrm.org

March of Dimes Birth Defects Foundation
888-MO-DIMES
www.modimes.org

National Institute for Occupational Safety and Health
800-356-4674

Organization of Teratology Information Services (OTIS) Pregnancy Riskline
888-285-3410

VEGETARIANISM
Seventh-day Adventist Dietetic Association
714-793-8918

The Vegetarian Nutrition Dietetic Practice Group of the American Dietetic Association
800-877-1600
www.eatright.org

Vegetarian Resource Group
410-366-8343
www.vrg.org

PUBLICATIONS
Food Allergies by Merri Lou Dobler, M.S., R.D. The American Dietetic Association, 1991. ISBN 0-88091-096-8. Be sure to specify the ISBN number. This is a booklet.

Food Allergies by Celide Barnes Koerner, M.S., R.D. and Anne Munoz-Furlong. The American Dietetic Association, John Wiley & Sons, 1998. Part of the Nutrition Now series.

Making Food Healthy and Safe (for day care workers). Available from the National Maternal and Child Health Clearinghouse: 800-370-2943; *www.nih.gov/nichd.*

The Nursing Mother's Companion by Kathleen Huggins, R.N., M.S. Harvard Common Press, 1999.

Pregnancy Nutrition: Good Health for You and Your Baby by Elizabeth M. Ward. The American Dietetic Association, John Wiley & Sons, 1998. Part of the Nutrition Now series.

The School Food Allergy Program by Anne Munoz-Furlong. The Food Allergy Network. See *www.foodallergy.org* to purchase or to apply for a free kit.

Tyler's Honest Herbal by Steven Foster and Varro Tyler. Haworth Herbal Press, Binghamton, NY, 1999.

INDEX

The Everything®
Baby's First Year Book

By Teklas Nee

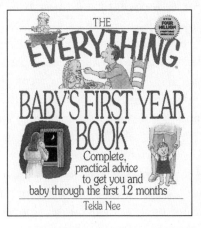

An indispensable guide to loving and nurturing a child during the most precious time of his or her life.

The first year of a newborn's life is a wonderful and challenging time for new and experienced parents alike. *The Everything® Baby's First Year Book* is a complete guide to surviving the first twelve months—from what to do when arriving home from the hospital with a newborn to handling feedings, bathing, and sleeping routines.

The Everything® Baby's First Year Book provides advice on every aspect of baby's physical, emotional, and social development. Written in an easy-to-follow style with a reassuring tone, this helpful book provides frustrated—and often sleep-deprived—parents with the quick answers they need to their toughest questions.

Featuring:
- Detailed suggestions on breastfeeding and bottle-feeding
- Soothing remedies for colic, teething, diaper rash, and other common problems
- Helpful recommendations on safe baby toys and games to play
- Useful advice on traveling with newborns and one-year-olds
- Important information on foods to avoid and general food preparation

8" x 9 ¼", 304 pages
2-color, with illustrations throughout
Trade Paperback
$12.95, ISBN: 1-58062-581-9

The Everything®
Toddler Book

By Linda Sonna, Ph.D.

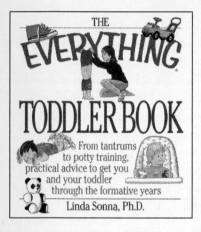

An indispensable guide to surviving the toddler years.

The toddler years can be a challenging time for both new and experienced parents. *The Everything® Toddler Book* is a complete guide to surviving these exciting and turbulent times when young, determined children begin to walk, talk, eat adult food, use a potty—and learn the art of refusal.

The Everything® Toddler Book provides professional advice on every aspect of physical, emotional, and social development. Written in an easy-to-follow style with a reassuring tone, this helpful book provides frustrated—and often sleep-deprived—parents the quick answers they need to their toughest questions.

Includes:
- Great meals toddlers will actually sit still for and eat
- Soothing remedies for teething and other common problems
- Helpful advice on the best toys and games to play
- Travel tips—from restaurants to airplane vacations
- Special concerns regarding siblings, both older and younger
- Hints for tackling the challenges of potty training

8" x 9 ¼", 304 pages
Two-color, with illustrations throughout
Trade Paperback
$12.95, ISBN: 1-58062-592-4

Available wherever books are sold.
For more information, or to order, call 800-872-5627
or visit *www.adamsmedia.com*
Adams Media Corporation, 57 Littlefield Street, Avon, MA 02322